Living Thin

Living Young

Living Thin
An Attitude — Not a Diet

Living Young
An Attitude, Not an Age

SYLVIA M. GOLDMAN
Foreword By Albert Ellis, Ph.D.

Glenbridge Publishing Ltd.

Illustrations
Patricia Hobbs

Copyright © 2000 by Sylvia M. Goldman

Published by Glenbridge Publishing Ltd.
19923 E. Long Ave.
Aurora, Colorado 80016

Library of Congress Catalog Card Number: LC 00-100347

International Standard Book Number: 0-944435-49-1

10   9   8   7   6   5   4   3   2   1

Contents

Foreword by Albert Ellis, Ph.D. vii

Preface ix

Acknowledgments xiii

1 Become Your Own Nutritionist,
Your Own Therapist. 1

2 Living Thin Above the Neck 26

3 Step Into My Classroom and Let's Get Started 61

4 Living Thin Below the Neck 97

5 Your Health, Living Young, and Exercise 135

6 Living Thin on the Run 188

7 Living Assertively Is An Art Form . . .
Learn To Do It With Style 200

8 Getting Started. 242

9 Nuts, Bolts, and "Staying Tuned" 249

Notes 289

Bibliography 291

Index 293

To Garth

without whom it would never have been written —
we did the first two chapters together, and that got me going.

Foreword

Sylvia M. Goldman's *Living Thin, Living Young* is a notable addition to the materials that tell you, the reader, how to effectively use Rational Emotive Behavior Therapy (REBT) with the problem of getting thin and staying that way. I originated REBT in January 1955, after I discovered that psychoanalysis and other forms of psychotherapy were woefully inefficient and helped little with overeating, procrastination, and other problems involving low frustration tolerance and self-downing. I therefore applied REBT to many practical problems of living, including love and sex relationships, business affairs, assertiveness training, and the disturbed feelings of anxiety, depression, anger, and self-pity.

About ten years after I originated REBT, other forms of Cognitive Behavior Therapy (CBT) followed — such as those of Aaron Beck, Donald Meichenbaum, and William Glasser. These psychotherapies show how people's emotional and behavioral problems can be most effectively tackled by showing how they use irrational beliefs to upset themselves and how they can employ a number of cognitive, emotive, and behavioral methods to change their dogmatic, grandiose "shoulds" and "musts" back into rational preferences. Today, REBT and CBT are perhaps the most widely used forms of therapy in the United States and Europe and are increasing in popularity. Many research studies have shown them to be quite efficient. REBT has produced several self-help books and tapes on dealing with eating problems, including my book, *The Art and Science of Rational*

Eating, my tape, I'd Like to Stop But . . . Overcoming Addictions, and Myles Faith's pamphlet, "Long Term Weight Management and Self-Acceptance."

Sylvia Goldman's *Living Thin, Living Young* is a clear and highly readable book that shows you how to apply the main principles of REBT to weight loss, low frustration tolerance, unassertiveness, lack of self-acceptance, and other important problems. It especially emphasizes the crucial element of motivation and tells you how to increase it. It gives many case studies of individuals whom Sylvia Goldman has helped over the years to live thin and be happy doing so. It deals with practical dieting issues in a non-fanatic manner. I cannot endorse its dieting rules, because that is not my field of expertise, but Sylvia presents them in a flexible, experimental manner that will help many people.

Try these principles. Really use its REBT methods of self-help to see how they work for you. The book makes no guarantees and offers no miracles, but it includes much valuable material that you may find potentially helpful.

Albert Ellis, Ph.D.
President, Albert Ellis Institute
for Rational Emotive Behavior Therapy

Preface

How You Will Benefit From Reading This Book

Living Thin is dedicated to all the "DCs" anywhere and everywhere who allow their "stinking thinking" habits to stop them from reaching a much desired goal of healthy and permanent weight loss.

What is a DC? A DC is a difficult customer — individuals who want what they want on their terms. They want a form of magic that simply doesn't exist. A DC is intimately connected to the garbage in his or her head, to negative messages that say, "I know what to do, I just don't feel like doing it." *Living Thin — Living Young* will teach DCs how to get rid of the garbage in their heads by having them tell themselves repeatedly, "I don't have to FEEL LIKE DOING IT, I just have to DO it."

In other words, Dr. Albert Ellis's REBT (Rational Emotive Behavior Therapy), which is the foundation of *Living Thin — Living Young*, will help you cope with daily stress so that you don't fall apart when life rains on your parade. The success of my Living Thin Program is based on sound thinking habits that will help you find the simple solution you want so you can meet your goals. Rational thinking makes Living Thin a fringe benefit of better physical and emotional health.

We're not talking about the kind of stress that merely involves a busy schedule. Nor are we talking about a life free from stress of any kind. The enjoyment of planning to attend a much anticipated event or party, traveling to new and exciting places, beginning an exciting, challenging job that involves meeting deadlines — all of these experiences carry the good stress that is part of enjoying the good life. I agree with Helen Gurley Brown's contention that "automobiles never driven are stress-free, but their batteries die."

Our goal is not being totally stress free or else our lives would resemble a piece of limp asparagus. We are talking about the kind of stress Dr. Marc Weinberg, of Sarasota, Florida, refers to when he says, "If a stress response is chronic, its constant presence will, in time, wear down the body's immune system."

Not only are you going to Get Thin and Live Thin, you will be provided with coping strategies in this book for dealing with the "upsettedness" that makes change so difficult. Important to remember: NO ONE CAN DIE FOR YOU AND NO ONE CAN DIET FOR YOU.

You will learn that the magic you want lies within yourself and how to use that unique magic for your own goals and aspirations. You will learn to accept yourself "as is," to work with yourself, with your foibles and failings. And, as Shakespeare warns us, to avoid making comparisons.

What does it mean to have the courage to accept yourself "as is"? If you have a compulsive personality, you will be able to tell yourself that it is OK to be compulsive. In fact, you will learn how to goof off and still be in charge, to have an occasional binge (which is all you want anyway), and still be in charge of your weight. When you insist on perfection, you may create a form of stress that creates the anxiety that drives you to the cookie jar. I will be at your side every moment and help you create a lifestyle tailored to your eating and living habits.

Each person is unique. That statement gives me the courage to be who I am, with all my failings, and to remember that, because I am unique, there is no one solution that will work for all of us any more than one eyeglass prescription will suit everyone.

In summary you will learn:

- Guidelines — a set of simple rules for rational thinking that will guide your life — NO MATTER WHAT HAPPENS
- How to accept yourself — the good, the bad, and the ugly
- How to eliminate the need for perfection
- Why and how being assertive is so vital to success in any area
- What being assertive really means in terms of your emotional health
- The role of motivation in your life — where it comes from and how to keep it
- Suggestions for getting started in terms of calories and food
- How to have an eating binge without gaining weight
- Specific guidelines for creating PERMANENT CONNEC-TIONS that will help you to keep the weight off

Acknowledgments

Dr. Albert Ellis
Whose philosophy and support guaranteed the success of my program. My thanks to him for his support and willingness to endorse my work.

Jane Carr
Who designed the *Living Thin* logo and other drawings.

Jane Gugel
Whose initial editing made me realize that my work looked appealing — good enough to make a book.

Louis Lasky
My educational mentor, who helped me realize life's real adventure lies in learning — whatever the topic — from growing pansies to healthy weight control. The "joy" of learning he taught me eventually led to this book.

Drs. Norma Hauserman-Campbell and Jack Osman
Who helped me design my Living Thin Program.

Rick Lamport and Dr. Stephen Goldstein
Whose enthusiasm for my manuscript finally resulted in my reaching a publisher, introduced to me by Nicci Kobritz.

Dr. Harry Klinefelter
Whose support in my early years was invaluable.

Barbara Galler
Whose joy and appreciation for the program resulted in the formation of a scholarship for teenagers.

And to the many individuals who took and endorsed my program whose encouragement kept me moving forward: among them Charlotte and Albert Kaufman, Dr. David Hungerford, Dr. Alan Davis, Rabbi Mark Loeb, Achsah O'Donovan, George Gephardt and so many others.

1

Become Your Own Nutritionist, Your Own Therapist

I am *not* a dietitian, *not* a physician, *not* a therapist, so how come I have the *chutzpah* to teach others — and you in particular? What you are about to learn is the result of my own personal problem with weight control coupled with what my students have taught me about "TAKING IT OFF AND KEEPING IT OFF" without deprivation and without having to give up all of my favorite foods. With the help of professionals in the fields of nutrition, exercise, and mental health I designed the **LIVING THIN PROGRAM** and have been teaching it successfully for more than eighteen years; I continue to teach it as of this writing to men, women, and teenagers.

When several of my board members assured me that what I had designed so many years ago is a program that is so much more than learning how to "take it off and keep it off" but actually a design for preventive health, I knew it was time for a book!

I hear you loud and clear . . . you've heard it before . . . sounds too good to be true! Well, I refuse to apologize. This time you've hit the JACKPOT! You will learn how to be in charge of your weight problem in just nine chapters — providing you do what I tell you to do!

Does that sound like a contradiction? You may think you already know how to be in charge. How is doing what I tell you going to "put *you* in charge"? And the answer is, you will be *motivated* to DO the things you know how to do. You may emerge at the end of this book with a lifestyle that not only helps you lose weight but will become a blueprint for better health. Suspend your disbelief for the time it takes you to digest this book. Follow my instructions; this program works! I'll make a BELIEVER out of you!

Let me begin by explaining how the Living Thin Program began. Then, later in this chapter, I will introduce you to a variety of issues that are closely related to changing the way you think and eat.

> ## Don't Wait For Life to Happen — MAKE IT HAPPEN!

You will also learn how to identify and find solutions to roadblocks that have your name on them — roadblocks that interfere with change. So sit back and enjoy for now. Change comes later.

How I Found Out That Diets Don't Work — and What Does Work

My husband and I were very typical of our generation of comfortable, slightly overweight suburbanites. We worked hard at everything on our own *but* losing weight. As a matter of fact our favorite vacation spots were the many spas around the country.

Those elegant, stringent, resort-like places offered us a charming staff, brief physical exams, tasty but small amounts of food, and an opportunity to have it all by leaving a big check at the front desk! We left each time 10-15 pounds thinner, but within six months to a year the weight was back on. Of course, back to the spa we went again and again.

In between these visits to the spa I tried controlling my weight with every new fad diet that came along. One of my favorites was the Banana and Skim Milk Diet. You could have four bananas and four glasses of skim milk per day. Sure it worked to take off a few pounds, but as soon as I went back to my regular foods, the pounds came back. I didn't realize that I was consuming only 800 calories a day!

Oh, I forgot to tell you, I smoked a pack of cigarettes a day, which gave me automatic portion control. The day I decided to give up smoking, was I in big trouble! Realizing the health dangers associated with smoking, I wouldn't let myself return to cigarettes even though the weight began piling on. I panicked, tried all my old quick remedies, but nothing worked!

I was so obsessed with losing weight I would have sold my mother's diamond wedding ring for the answer to my problem. The year was 1975 and I did what so many others did — joined a local franchise of a national diet group and went to a meeting. There I sat, hoping I would find the solutions to losing weight. But what did I find? A great recipe for cheesecake and a bunch of ladies with big behinds sharing dessert recipes that they swore could make you thin!

Right away I knew this was a no-go. More than ten years earlier, in the early '60s, as a result of a unique learning experience, I had started my own school for adults called Adventures in Learning and became passionate about the joy of learning. Having become a snob about education, I could readily see there would be little learning at the weekly diet meetings. I would merely continue to be a supervised marionette with someone

┌─────────────────┐
│   │
│ WEIGHT LOSS IS │
│ SCIENTIFIC.   │
│   │
└─────────────────┘

else pulling my strings and not explaining the food choices on my plan, which matched everyone else's plan too! One meeting was enough! I ran home and begged everyone I knew for a name of anyone who could help me. The first name I received was that of a private dietitian nearby. Did I ever make a beeline for her! She taught me a simple solution to my problem. She said it over and over again: *Weight loss is scientific, like the sun that rises in the east and sets in the west.* She believed in the old adage: It's better to teach you how to fish than to hand you the fish, which is how she helped me understand the basic components of weight loss and to tailor them to my needs, not my mother-in-law's, not my neighbor's, not my sister-in-law's — especially not my sister-in-law's!

You don't have to be a rocket scientist to learn the basic premise of weight loss. To lose weight, a person must simply expend more calories of energy than he or she takes in through eating. To keep it off, the scales of intake and output must be balanced over the long haul.

The simplicity of what the dietitian taught me enraged me, because it made me realize that I, like thousands of others had been HAD — first, by a society that insists how unhealthy and unattractive it is to be overweight, and second by an industry that manipulates people by capitalizing on their strong desire to lose weight while taking advantage of their need to have someone do it for them.

The message became glaringly obvious: weight loss was and is BIG BUSINESS! Instead of educating people and teaching them how to reach their ideal weight and become fit for life, the weight loss industry in all too many cases sells quick-fix, temporary, one-size-fits-all solutions for getting thin. The diet/ weight loss industry never was, and never will be, education oriented. After all, there's no money in education. Long-term success with weight loss means death for the weight loss industry. Weight loss is a failure business because a dieter's long-term success would mean no repeat business. This would be a problem when their next month's rent is due.

So many books and articles about weight loss have appeared, but as weight loss programs proliferated, the problem of obesity escalated. When they found a cure for polio, we stopped hearing about the problem! What does that say about weight loss? The weight loss industry hasn't found the cure! Maybe it doesn't want to find the cure!

I became convinced the key to permanent weight loss is education. For all these reasons there was born within me a strong desire to offer a sound,

> **People of America: The greatest threat to the survival of you and your children is not some terrible nuclear weapon. It is what you are going to eat from your dinner plate tonight!**
>
> David Reuben, M.D.

scientific, honest, and easy-to-learn weight loss program through my school. If an individual can learn how to play golf, how to play bridge, how to make love, why not learn how to take weight off and keep it off healthily and permanently? So I turned to the many experts who had participated in my school for adult education. It was through my contact with Dr. Kenneth

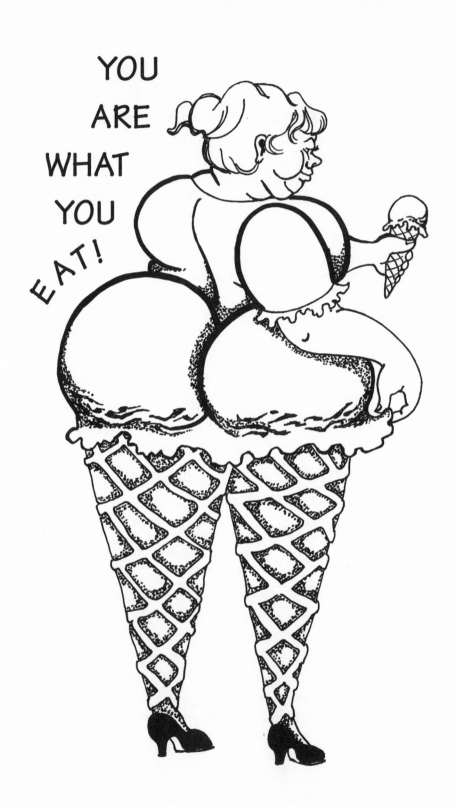

Shaw, an invaluable advisor and currently chancellor of Syracuse University, that I met Dr. Jack Osman.

Osman, a health scientist and a published writer and expert in the field of weight loss, had just finished researching and writing a book, *Thin From Within*. He agreed to bring his knowledge to my students at Adventures in Learning, and I took on the marketing of the course. Many people succeeded in losing weight in this course, but getting thin didn't seem to be the hard part. It was keeping it off that was the trick. The goal was to stay at that desired weight!

For two years Adventures in Learning offered the course. In spite of Dr. Osman's sincerity and commitment, the course was not working — people were not maintaining their weight loss. In spite of my daily calls and close attention to each client, all I heard were excuses for not following the program.

Classes were held every Monday evening. I vividly recall one Monday when two students, who where taking the course together, approached me after the first class. Each one had at least 50 or 60 pounds to lose.

"Sylvia, we have a conflict in our schedule. We can't be here next Monday evening. We have a dinner party!" one explained.

"YOU ARE GOING TO A DINNER PARTY?" I said disbelievingly. "Let me have the address. Look at me and look at you. I'll go to the dinner party and you come here!"

So many excuses . . . Any excuse would do! It became painfully clear that this program, like so many others, was failing too. I had a hard time understanding why.

Once again I went to see Dr. Shaw. He introduced me to Dr. Norma Hauserman-Campbell, a psychologist trained in REBT (Rational Emotive Behavior Therapy) and currently director of The Norbel School in Baltimore, Maryland. She explained that weight loss was a problem that existed above the neck, a "head problem," so to speak, and unless my students could learn how to cope with the daily issues that upset them, there would be little chance of weight loss — especially long-term weight loss. **Something finally made sense!**

Through Dr. Hauserman-Campbell I met Dr. Albert Ellis, the father of cognitive-behavior therapy and the founder, director, and president of the world famous Albert Ellis Institute headquartered in New York City. Dr. Ellis tells us that we upset ourselves with our MUSTS and SHOULDS, while making unreasonable demands on ourselves and others. We are all born with a natural propensity for "stinking thinking." He is convinced that we can all become more rational thinkers and indeed become our own therapists.

At long last I had found the key, the missing ingredient! I redesigned my program to thoroughly incorporate Dr. Ellis's philosophy and in so doing to give students the tools and skills for self-discipline that were missing in their lives. The addition of REBT was the guarantee, the "insurance," that the success they enjoyed in the classroom would continue.

Word Gets Out

Because of my unique approach to weight loss, the Living Thin Program attracted the attention of the Baltimore medical community. This was not a medical community to be taken lightly! Among the eminent physicians who supported my program was Dr. Harry Klinefelter, on the faculty of Johns Hopkins School of Medicine. Known throughout the world because of his involvement with the identification of a rare chromosomal abnormality afflicting males (known as Klinefelter's syndrome), Klinefelter became an active spokesperson for the Living Thin Program, which further contributed to its success.

Not only did Dr. Klinefelter become a medical advisor but also a close friend. Our monthly lunches kept me current on the latest findings on the connection between health and weight. Thus, my trio of advisors became Osman in the field of nutrition, Klinefelter in the field of medicine, and Hauserman-Campbell in the field of psychology.

All the information I'm sharing with you is a compilation and synthesis of the many books I've read, the experts I've consulted, and the students I've taught over the years.

What's It All About?

So why don't diets work? Why do we lose and gain, lose and gain? Why is losing weight and keeping it off *so* tough? Why do statistics tell us that Americans are getting fatter with each new advancement in weight loss? What are the problems? What is it *really* all about?

It's about people wanting magic — about people wanting to fall asleep overweight and wake up thin. It's about a society that insists on searching for EASY ANSWERS — about physicians who don't even understand the problem. It's about commercializing the problem. It's about others who are willing to delude the public into thinking that "DIETS" work! It's about being told that "THIN IS IN!" while we are constantly being bombarded with "goodies." It's about lifestyles filled with stress that drive us to the cookie jar. It's about thinking we can do it with

> You are not overweight because you have a glandular imbalance or because your parents were fat or because you're unlucky in love. You are overweight because YOU EAT TOO MUCH!

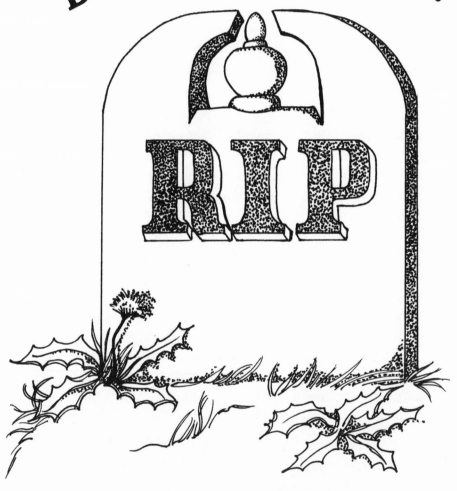

pills and powders that eventually make us fat and very often sick! It's about an unwillingness to grow up and assume responsibility for our health. Are you ready? Only you can make that decision!

Loving Yourself Tough
Is What Living Thin Is All About

Living Thin, Living Young is about **Loving Yourself Tough**. What does this mean? It means caring enough about yourself to make you do hard things. Loving Yourself Tough means caring enough about yourself to make you overcome the inertia that afflicts almost all of us. Best of all, Loving Yourself Tough means that you *can* have it all. You *can* find a way of eating and exercising that is satisfying and compatible with your tastes and lifestyle. By Loving Yourself Tough you can learn to be in charge of how much or how little you weigh. You *can learn* to be in control of yourself emotionally, mentally, and physically.

The rational thinking tools that I'm giving you in this book will make it easier to do the things you want to do. You will learn how to deal with the following issues the Living Thin way and Love It:

- What motivation is and how to hold on to it. How to get rid of all your excuses — including the one you're thinking of at this very moment
- How assertion, passivity, aggression, and approval seeking are all connected to change, especially in the area of weight loss
- How to find a way of eating and exercising that is moderately comfortable for you
- How to design your own personal blueprint for self-maintenance

Don't stop! Don't be overwhelmed! Now I hear you loud and clear. Maybe you've tried it all before. But this time I will be with you *all the way*, and I promise you'll love the journey.

So Diets Don't Work . . . What *Does* Work?

In the area of weight loss much has been written and rewritten about the ill effects of dieting. A dangerous consequence of dieting is referred to as "yo-yoing." The yo-yo effect happens simply because a low calorie diet slows down the metabolism. When you return to your old eating habits, you find to your dismay that you now need to eat even less then you did prior to the diet, simply because you "dieted."

The biggest complaint that I hear from my students is that they have been on and off more diets than they care to remember. You know the ones we're talking about. They are all out there, ready to take your money, and they will continue to multiply as long as you keep looking for easy answers, answers that never deal with the very behaviors that got you fat in the first place. You may have also picked up this book saying, *"Here we go again."* But remember, I told you that Living Thin is a lifestyle, not a diet. It's true. Slow, steady weight loss is what *staying power* is all about.

All right, I let it slip. You are going to learn about staying power. Staying power requires you to deal with your LFT — Low Frustration Tolerance. LFT simply is a low tolerance for being frustrated. Living Thin, Living Young allows you to change your bad eating habits into good ones while you continue to lose weight.

> **TODAY, I WILL NOT SHOULD ON MYSELF!**

Living Thin is not just a solution! This program teaches you to overcome your LFT, increases your staying power, and will increase your ability to forego the need for instant gratification involved in unhealthy and quick weight loss programs.

Reading Alone Won't Work!

Let's talk for a moment about really knowing how to do something. You don't really know something until you can act on it. A good analogy would be learning a new word or language. You don't "own" a word until you can use it. It's the same with information. You don't own the information until you use it. Knowing isn't good enough. Knowledge alone is valueless.

Knowing is doing, said the great American philosopher and educator, John Dewey. You need to get out of that chair and put the words you're reading — the whole Living Thin Program — into action. Just thinking about them won't wash. Reading may sharpen your intellect, but it won't dull your appetite.

Go Public!

The more you talk about any topic the more chance you have for success. For many years I taught three classes a week, each class containing thirty people or more. These were nine-week courses. At the conclusion of the first class I turned to the group and my question was always, "How many of you are going to tell others about your being on the Living Thin Program?" Rarely did a hand go up. Instead, they freely admitted how ashamed they would be for someone to learn that they were *once more* involved in a weight loss program — especially one costing $395. My response was, "I promise you will fail."

Why did I say this? Was I being cruel? No, not at all. Experience has taught me that when your friends, family, and co-workers know you're actively trying to lose weight, you are more motivated to achieve that goal. Let me give you an example of how it works. You go out with a few friends and everyone orders apple pie with cinnamon-vanilla ice cream — your favorite. Secretly you tell yourself how fortunate — or wise — you were to have concealed your involvement with Living Thin. You've now given yourself permission to go full speed ahead. Your goose is cooked, only now it's apple pie à la mode.

My advice is Go Public! Tell people what you're trying to accomplish. Suppose you're at a dinner party. Someone serves the same apple pie à la mode, but this time you look the person on your right or left in the eye — friend or foe, doesn't matter — and say, *"Apple pie à la mode is my most favorite dish, but for medical reasons I'm not allowed to eat any at this time,"* or you can use any other excuse of your choosing. If you're willing to make that statement, I promise you will not eat any of that dessert. You WILL NOT make a liar out of yourself!

Self-Acceptance and Commitment

Now let's talk about self-acceptance and commitment. For change to happen you need to do it for the right reason — because YOU want it. Not for your doctor, not for your friend, not for anybody! And it's okay to be overweight! It's not against the law. When you're ready for a change, you'll know it.

If you're ready to make a commitment, then by all means make one that works! Here's an example of what I mean by a commitment that works. Let's assume that you've decided to read *Living Thin, Living Young* on Monday nights. If you are a surgeon, you simply don't operate on Monday night because Monday night is your night to Live Thin. If you are pregnant, you don't have your baby on Monday night. Monday night is your night to Live Thin.

Without a strong, powerful commitment you haven't a chance! You have the power to create your own mental environment that will reinforce your commitment. Be strong. Be decisive. It doesn't make sense to make commitments we don't honor. When your behavior fails to match your so-called stated goals in life, the message is loud and clear: YOU DON'T WANT IT ENOUGH, AND IT WON'T HAPPEN!

Attitudes, Attitudes, Attitudes

> *People are disturbed not by things, but by the view they take of them.*
> —EPICTETUS, 1ST CENTURY A.D.

Feelings, thoughts, and behaviors are connected. Your feelings do not come from the happening, they come from what you choose to tell yourself about any situation, and that means that what you choose to tell yourself is a choice! Whenever you find yourself faltering, hesitating as you move toward a goal, remember, you CAN choose thoughts that will give you motivation to continue in the right direction. Suppose I am exercising, using portion control, but the scale refuses to budge. I can choose to tell myself this is futile, useless, a waste of my time and energy, and that I may as well give up. Or, I can follow Sylvia's advice and look for the causes, which could easily be something as simple as a water retention problem caused by sodium consumption, causing true fat loss to be masked on the scale.

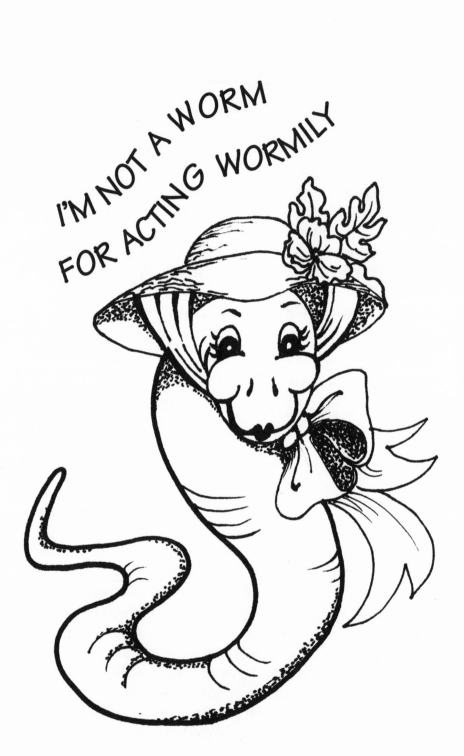

I KNOW WHAT TO DO, SO WHY DON'T I DO IT?

You know what to do, but you still don't do it! Why? Because you don't feel like doing it. Right? You're not alone. I have heard this complaint for twenty years. My response is always the same: "YOU DON'T HAVE TO FEEL LIKE DOING IT. YOU JUST HAVE TO DO IT!" I hear you. You don't feel like doing it because *"doing it"* means developing a new habit, and that *is* hard to do! It *is* hard, but not *too* hard. You have three choices: 1) move toward changing the habit; 2) refuse to change — keep the status quo; and 3) wail and whine. If you are committed to change, then *not* doing it is harder. Why not harness your energy for change? You need to be sure, however, to pinpoint the habit you want to change. With Living Thin you will develop an acute awareness of these unhelpful habits.

> I don't have to FEEL like doing it; I just have to DO it!

Another problem that gets in the way of change is denial. Overweight people are experts at denial. Let me tell you about Mildred. She was a student of mine who always came to class a little earlier than everyone else. She was the first to weigh in and always seemed to be happy to assist me with classroom duties before anyone appeared. Of course I attributed her early arrivals to her enthusiasm for the program. One evening Mildred, caught in traffic, arrived at class later than usual. As she was preparing to weigh in, she whispered in my ear, "Sylvia, please don't let anyone else in line see how much I weigh." My reply to this request is always the same: "They don't have to see the scale to learn how much you weigh. All they have to do is look at you." In spite of this pointed comment, Mildred kept telling herself that no one could really see how much she weighed.

My mother could fit comfortably in a size 20 but never bought any piece of clothing larger than a 16. She'd rather take the garment to a seamstress for alterations than admit she was a size 20. Very often we can't correct a problem unless we're ready to recognize the problem and give it credence. Facing the truth about your habits is the beginning of freeing yourself from that habit. Bad habits are roadblocks to change. See if the following roadblocks have your name on them!

Roadblock #1: Low Frustration Tolerance

We need to deal with our LFT, Low Frustration Tolerance — our need for immediate gratification. Babies need to have what they want when they want it. Adults are supposed to know better. Changes to eating and lifestyle habits need to be made slowly and gradually if they are to last. Your LFT undermines your commitment by pushing you to avoid doing anything that's unpleasant or uncomfortable. You say to yourself, "I shouldn't have to do it. I'd rather do without it. It's not worth it. It's not only hard, it's too hard!" It's also important to remember that to achieve a desirable solution you always have to include some inconvenience and discomfort. So it's tough and SO WHAT! Being unhealthy, waiting to have a heart attack is also unpleasant. Catch yourself when you start to say, "I don't feel like doing the things that I need to do!"

> It's never
> TOO HARD,
> it's just HARD!

and change the message to, *"I don't have to feel like doing them, I just have to do them and I'll begin to feel better about doing them after I begin enjoying the results. But there will be no re-sults unless I DO the things I don't feel like doing. I don't have to like it, I just have to do it. I can stand being inconvenienced. I AM NOT A BABY. Babies can't wait, but I can."*

You can overcome your LFT by practicing compromise, ne-gotiation, and moderation the Living Thin way.

Roadblock #2: Garbage in Your Head

The garbage in your head interferes with your learning. The garbage in your head stops you from thinking about what you are going to read in this book. The garbage tells you that you *already* know it all! Now you may know a lot, but you don't know it all or you wouldn't have bought this book, so why get into a power struggle with the very person who is trying to help you. Let's get rid of your "stinking thinking" and get down to the business of Living Thin. Not just Getting Thin. Getting Thin is a BIG NOTHING!

Roadblock #3: Boredom and Fatigue

Both of these conditions will absolutely erode your motiva-tion to make changes and adopt new habits. Develop a keen awareness about these problems. When you are tired, avoid overeating; rest instead. Fatigue is only cured with sleep and rest, *not* food. Boredom is only cured with planned activities. Make a list and force yourself to become a participant.

Roadblock #4: Portion Control

The secret to portion control lies in developing good eating habits so you are never *too* hungry. Good eating habits is a term

Garbage in the head

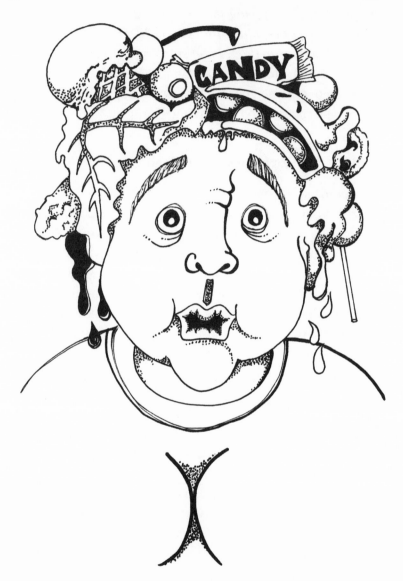

Garbage is a collection of preconceived ideas about nutrition, about life that interferes with change. The garbage in your head interferes with your hearing the information that will help you!

that refers to the food choices we make and how we choose to make them. Take Al for instance. Al is a very busy stockbroker with a very large portfolio and demanding clients. He eats out at the best restaurants New York has to offer at least three times a week. Al habitually skips breakfast on the days that he "power lunches" with his clients and always enters the restaurant with the idea of eating light.

However, by the time Al actually gets past that first martini he is so hungry that he can only think BIG! The decision to eat light is gone, and the unplanned and uncontrolled lunch has become the replacement. Al could have been in control and had his small lunch; he only needed to have a plan and never skip a meal!

> # We're digging our graves with our teeth!
> The Nutrition Revolution

Roadblock #5: Poor Food Choices

Nutrition occurs at the cell level. Everything we eat affects the 60 trillion cells in our bodies. The American public consumes about 75 percent of its diet in fats, sugars, salt, and alcohol — garbage foods. We are the sum total of all our cells. Our cells cooperate with one another. The sugars, greases, salts, alcohol that we choose to consume affects our cells. It's like injecting one home in the neighborhood with a form of poison gas, and that home affects the entire neighborhood. A rotten diet will affect my entire body, especially my vulnerable cells.

Here's an example I've used over the years. In my first class session I ask, "Anybody here eat potato chips?" Nine out of ten people say yes. I hold up a potato chip and say: "Before it was a potato chip it was a slice of potato. If we go to a factory that makes potato chips, we'll see the slicing is done by machine. After it's sliced, it's then inundated with oil. How clean is that oil? We'll never know. Then it's rolled in salt and packaged. You may have it with a cocktail or with a chicken salad sandwich, but you'll certainly be eating more than one potato chip. The salt ensures that. Ask yourself, 'What happens to the oil and the salt after I swallow it?' How do you think your body feels about ingesting the oil and the salt? Do you get rid of it immediately by elimination? Absolutely not. The oil and salt become very friendly and begin visiting our 60 trillion cells." Think about my potato chip story the next time you're about to swallow one.

> Eat as much as you like, just don't swallow.

Roadblock #6: Insufficient Activity

The human body is designed for activity, and we know that muscles atrophy without use. We've heard this for years. "Use it or lose it." The same principle applies to all bodily functions. Moderate exercise leads to improved circulation, which is the basis of health.

Okay, you've heard all this before. You're weary, tired, jaded from reading and hearing about the benefits of exercise. You avoid exercise because you don't FEEL like exercising. I know what you're telling yourself and how your thinking stops you from exercising.

Consider Jane, a diet dropout. Sure she lost 25 pounds, but they were slowly returning when her friend recommended the

Living Thin Program to her. Wailing and whining about how she hated to do any extra activity in her all-too-busy day, Jane proceeded to get into a power struggle

> **Heart Disease Begins in Your Stomach.**

over adding a few minutes of physical activity daily. She refrained from exercise and watched her weight creep back on. By the time she returned to Living Thin all but 5 of her 25 pounds had returned. Desperate and willing finally to follow the program as suggested, she gave up her power struggle and increased her activity with a 15-minute walk daily. Without changing her food plan she was able to walk off those extra pounds within several weeks.

Roadblock #7: Fear of Planning

I hear you again. You say, "There is no way I want the responsibility of making a daily plan. I don't want to be boxed in!" The truth is PLANNING SETS YOU FREE.

Planning gives you the freedom to change; your plan is not set in concrete. Planning will give you benefits — advantages you could never have when others do your planning for you. You will make the choices and you will be in charge. When we allow others to make our choices, we can all too easily become dependent. PLANNING FREES YOU FROM MAKING MOMENT-TO-MOMENT DECISIONS. Without a plan you may be rethinking, changing your mind all day. "Hmmm, that brownie smells great; maybe I'll have a piece . . . but maybe I shouldn't . . . so many calories." This type of thinking and agonizing takes up a lot of time. By making a plan in advance you are making it easier to make decisions. Whether you give up the brownie or eat it is *not* the issue, the issue is BEING IN CHARGE. By having a plan, I am making my own choices instead of letting it happen.

Another plus for planning applies especially to difficult situations like weekends, parties, and vacations. The secret lies in having a plan that will provide you with eating choices that

> MY PROBLEM IS EMOTIONAL. WHENEVER I GET UPSET, I TURN TO A COOKIE . . . .

are moderately satisfying and will help you avoid hunger. When you allow yourself to feel "hunger pangs," you are at the mercy of your appetite. It's so easy when you have a plan. Planning puts you in charge, and isn't that what you really want?

Roadblock #8: Emotional Eating

For an overeater, using food for the wrong reasons is a natural and predictable response to a negative emotion. Searching for relief from negativity such as depression, anxiety, boredom, loneliness, or frustration is normal. The alcoholic turns to alcohol, the druggie to drugs, and the overeater to food. I want you to become your own therapist, so that when negative feelings overtake you, you will have the tools and the skills for reducing, diffusing, or even eliminating them.

Summary

You now have a thumbnail sketch of why the weight loss business doesn't help you lose weight. There are no easy answers to losing weight, only simple solutions. If you do what I tell you to do, you will very soon find a formula that will tell you almost precisely how much you can eat and how much activity you will need to get the results that you want. Your decisions can then be based on sound information centered around you. Learn how your body works. Be in charge.

I love Living Thin because I know exactly the kind of choices that suit me. I've done my homework. If the scale goes up, I know what to do about it, and I can do it without being hungry — best of all without giving up my manhattan cocktail!

> If you want to look young and thin, hang out around old, fat people . . . .

2

Living Thin Above the Neck

"Disturbed feelings about eating can be traced to irrational, inflexible, absolutist thinking."
— ALBERT ELLIS, PH.D.,
THE ART & SCIENCE OF RATIONAL EATING

Living Thin Rationally in an Irrational World

Am I to believe that controlling my emotional responses will keep me slender? Does that mean all "cool cats" are slender, and all "overweights" are "hyper" and out of control? Yes and No. There are no black and white answers, especially about how individuals lose weight. However, after many years of teaching, observing, and counseling, I do believe that clear thinking and giving up overreacting to daily problems that often cause you to become unduly depressed, angry, frustrated, anxious — whatever the negative feeling — *will* help you to avoid or at least make it easier for you to *do* hard things, such as giving up noshing just for the momentary joy of noshing.

When I am unduly upset, turning to food for relief is natural. When an alcoholic is upset, he turns to alcohol — a druggie to drugs — but a foodaholic's problem is more difficult. A person can survive without alcohol or drugs, but a person cannot survive without food. For all these reasons *becoming your own therapist* will help you develop strong insides — emotional muscle — and make "taking and keeping it off" much easier.

When I began teaching rational thinking, my students' successes increased significantly, as did their ability to maintain their weight loss. For these reasons, I am now convinced that becoming your own therapist has a major role in — is in fact crucial to — making lifestyle changes.

Learning to be in control of my emotional responses to life gives me an inner strength, and it's the same strength that helps me say "no" to a cookie. It gives me the resolve to talk to myself — to teach and train myself. It hardens my attitude. It makes it easier for me to do the things I need to do.

> I have talked with Sylvia Goldman and listened to some of her main presentations of the theory and practice of Rational Emotive Behavior Therapy (REBT). In the course of investigating the REBT aspects of her Living Thin Seminars, I have found that she understands REBT very well, is an excellent teacher of it, uses it effectively with people who have emotional problems about maintaining their weight loss, and helps them in other important ways.
>
> Albert Ellis, Ph.D.

Now, let's learn more about rational thinking, Rational-Emotive Behavior Therapy and its founder, Dr. Albert Ellis.

REBT's Founder

Dr. Albert Ellis will go down in behavioral history with Sigmund Freud and B.F. Skinner. Over more than five decades Ellis has built a significant public and professional reputation by his scientific achievements in the field of psychology. Over the years, he has been recognized and awarded high honors from many professional organizations and has been named Distinguished Psychologist, Scientific Researcher, and Distinguished Psychological Practitioner by the American Society of Psychotherapists. As a result of his work, there are now REBT institutes throughout the world.

REBT in a Nutshell

When it first appeared in 1961, *A Guide to Rational Living,* by Albert Ellis and Richard Harper, was one of the first books by reputable, experienced psychotherapists that showed people how to deal with their own problems. It was a revolutionary approach. Ellis advocates that we learn to think for ourselves,

---

REBT: You upset yourself with your SHOULDS, MUSTS, "AWFULIZING." Give up Demanding, Insisting and "Musting." Change them to Desiring, Preferring and "IT WOULD BE NICE BUT IT'S NOT A MUST."

teaching us to identify, challenge, and block out old self-defeating behavioral patterns — in other words, how to be healthy thinkers.

Ellis tells us that our thoughts, feelings, and behaviors are connected. The thoughts I choose to have will influence to a great extent my feelings and my behavior. For example, I can choose to believe that I can overcome, can cope with, nearly all forms of adversity and, if I am willing to practice this style of thinking, my feelings and behaviors will begin matching my thoughts.

Ellis says we upset ourselves and create stress in our lives by demanding that people and life give us what we want on our own terms. In his writings, lectures, and tapes, Ellis demonstrates how we upset ourselves unnecessarily with our "shoulds," "musts," and "oughts." He suggests that we change our demands and say to ourselves, "It *would be* nice if my boss appreciated me, but I can stand it if he doesn't." In other words, we would be happier if we accepted the fact that we have control over the way we respond to others, to the world, and to ourselves; but we cannot control the way others behave or feel. It might be nice if, on occasion, we could control the attitudes and feelings of others, but we need to realize that we don't have that power.

Even more importantly, we need to realize that others have a *right* to behave differently. They have the right to be neurotic, to be selfish, and we don't have to like it or approve of it or even to accept it, but if we don't accept it, we're going to walk around upset most of the time because we have little or no control over the way others feel and behave.

Of course, we also have rights. We have the right to dislike the behavior of others. We have the right to try and change others. But we don't have the power to control what they do or say.

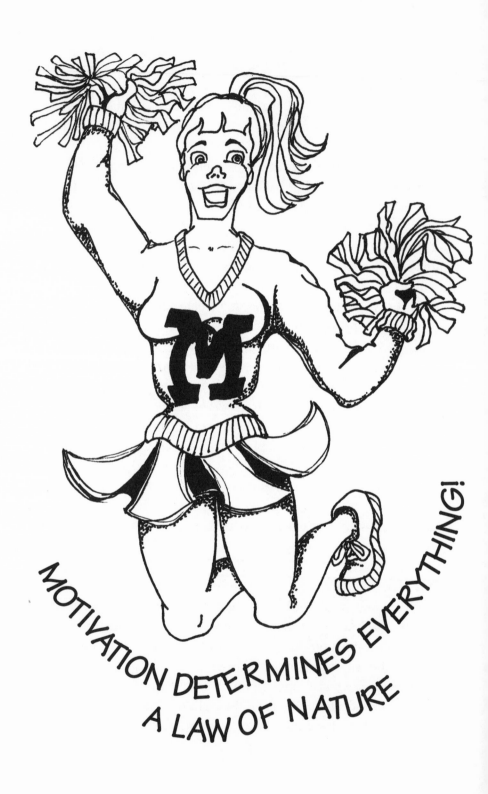

MOTIVATION DETERMINES EVERYTHING!
A LAW OF NATURE

REBT is a practical, action-oriented approach to coping with daily problems. Although people may be strongly influenced by events in their early lives, REBT does not spend years rehashing the past. The focus is mainly on the present — on changing currently held attitudes and behaviors that block us from achieving our goals.

Motivation

Change is impossible without motivation. There is no way you are going to do the things you need to do if you lack motivation. Anne is a young woman whose doctor insisted that she join my Living Thin group. Anne was 30 pounds overweight, depressed, and determined to avoid doing any of the things she was told to do.

"Anne, are you dating?" I asked her.

"No," she replied.

"How do you feel about that?"

"Well, I'm very picky. As a professional person, I'd like to find a doctor — and a tall one. (Anne is 5'9".)

It just so happens that there was a woman in the class whose son was tall, handsome, and a very successful cardiologist.

"Oh gee, I'd love to meet him. Will you introduce us?" Anne said.

But here's the hitch: the cardiologist only liked slender women. Do you think Ann had any problem losing weight after that? What does that tell you about motivation?

The better you feel about yourself, the more motivated you are to do hard things. Now let's talk about how to get the job done. We need to understand that **self-discipline** is not a dirty word.

Self-Discipline Is Not A Dirty Word

Let's face it. Self-discipline is the key, the magic that will give you what you want. To what avail to be intelligent, talented, if I don't have what it takes to make myself do the things I need to do to get what I want in life? How can I reach any goal or overcome obstacles? Or for our purposes, how can I say "no" to a piece of fried chicken or fried *anything* if I lack sufficient discipline?

So I love fried chicken, but my body doesn't love fried chicken or fried *anything*. And I know that eating anything fried is both unhealthy and makes weight loss more difficult. What's wrong with a piece of delicious chicken that has been roasted? Making that statement requires a form of self-discipline that is often missing in people who insist on looking for magic. They refuse to give up fried foods and they also want to lose weight. Their problem is grandiosity and entitlement.

This reminds me of a support group I was working with and one of its members, Sherri, a fashion consultant and a very stunning woman. I vividly recall her saying in this meeting, "I hear you loud and clear, Sylvia, but you don't understand. Sylvia, I know what you want me to do, but what you fail to understand is that when I go to a ball game, my idea of a good time is drinking beer and eating nachos all evening. And after a round of golf at the country club, my idea of fun is joining the group and having four or five cocktails."

> Some people regard discipline as a chore. For me, it is a kind of order that sets me free to fly.
>
> Julie Andrews

My response was, "Sounds like you're having a great time. What do you want from me?"

"You know what I want. I want to lose weight."

I then said, "Oh, I see. Your problem is a combination of grandiosity and entitlement. You want the world to make special rules for you. Elizabeth Taylor has tried and has never found anybody to make these special rules for her. If you find that person, I'd like to know about it — so would Elizabeth! The world knows how hard Elizabeth Taylor has tried to lose weight, and so far she hasn't succeeded. I'm afraid you won't either." But I have told you, over and over again, that weight loss is scientific. When you consume approximately 3,500 calories less than your body requires to maintain its present weight, your body will automatically drop a pound of fat.

Did Sherri like my message? No, of course not. But guess what? I saw her at the Food Fair with her husband a year later and she looked like a million — slender and confident. I approached her and said, "You look marvelous. How did you do it? You owe me an explanation."

"You know damn well what I did," she said, "I finally got the message."

What I'm saying to all you Sherries is once you get the message it's not that hard. To all you Sherries, you can have it all. It's so easy when you're willing to do your homework.

Thomas Edison said that genius is 10 percent inspiration and 90 percent perspiration. **In turn, weight loss is 10 percent the food and 90 percent your attitude.** Anyone reading this book is capable of achieving the stature and excitement that comes from being a disciplined person. Why not go for the long-term rather than the short-term solution for once? Believe me. It works!

Now let's discipline ourselves and examine a few common obstacles to self-discipline.

Low Frustration Tolerance: As we have shown, babies need to have what they want immediately. They are into short-range and immediate pleasures. For babies this approach is often healthy and necessary, but as adults these reasons no longer are valid. Getting what we want quickly is all too often the harmful way of satisfying our needs. *Taking things slowly and making gradual changes are the way to go.*

Refusing to Accept Reality: Before you can discipline yourself you need to be willing to accept the truth. Admitting the truth about ourselves is not easy. "Telling the truth" sounds like pie-in-the-sky moralizing, but without it, change cannot happen. The choice, as always, is yours. You must first recognize a problem before you can begin to change it. By insisting that things should not be a certain way, you are refusing to recognize that they *are* that way. So you do what you need to do or let it go. Repeat: DO WHAT YOU NEED TO DO OR LET IT GO.

Another choice is to wail and whine instead of "letting it go." Wailing and whining will not help you lose weight. It will help you alienate even your best friends. There are those who can eat as much as they wish and still be the lead in any fashion show. I know it seems unfair but so what! Life is unfair. But learning to accept that which you cannot change will make your job easier.

Boredom: Another hilltop climb in developing self-discipline skills is coping with boredom. Take Joan, for example. Throughout her school years Joan was charming, bright, witty, likable, but because she possessed so many natural attributes she rarely had to work hard to achieve a goal — until she left the classroom. She then discovered that boredom is very often part and parcel of achieving important goals, but she had little practice or experience dealing with boredom. Because she was so pleasure-loving, she refused to tolerate boredom. Joan simply failed to recognize and accept that boredom is a facet of almost any endeavor.

When Joan began gaining weight after having three children, she found, to her horror, that she was unable to lose this weight easily. She thought it was just too hard. She then joined several weight loss programs and would take it off but failed to keep it off — because she *dieted* instead of changing her lifestyle. Joan simply refused to recognize and accept that BOREDOM IS A FACET OF ALMOST ANY ENDEAVOR.

Joan says, "Counting calories is so boring."

"So is your big behind," I reply.

Joining program after program in the hope that someone else can do it for you is also boring. It is virtually impossible to do anything that you ordinarily enjoy without at times enduring some boredom. Getting started in nearly any venture can be boring, and SO WHAT! So it's boring.

Joan thought about my comments to her and instead of resenting them, returned to the next class and said, "I thought about it, and you're right. My big behind is boring. She went on to become one of the most successful students in the class.

Think of the consequences: the feeling of accomplishment when you feel better physically (more energy), emotionally, enjoying how you look in your clothes, or especially without your clothes! The time involved is so meager once you have some idea of how many calories you're eating. You are in charge! — a small price to pay for control. I've made counting calories so simple you will love the experience. In Chapter 4 you can look forward to counting calories Sylvia's way.

Guilt: Another obstacle is guilt. Losing weight is an area that is loaded with guilt feelings. You eat one cookie and feel bad all day for having been weak for a moment. Feeling guilty and full of self-reproach is a waste of time. If you allow yourself to feel that way for very long, you are likely to repeat the excess eating as your own neurotic way out of your dilemma.

Power Struggles: Even though Mary is desperately seeking a solution to her weight problem, when she's told what to do, she rebels and decides she is not going to do the very thing she needs to do. She resents having somebody telling her what to do. She wants to prove that the person giving her instructions can't boss her around. Mary comes to class for the purpose of being told what to do, but becomes angry when she is told — just another fine example of "stinking thinking." Instead, she could tell herself, "I came to find a solution to my problem. It doesn't make sense to get into a power struggle with the very person who is here to help me. I don't have to like her; I just have to do what she tells me to do."

Champion of Self-Discipline

In his book *How to Do What You Want To Do: The Art of Self-Discipline*, Dr. Paul Hauck relates a radio interview that demonstrates the power of self-discipline more clearly than any example I've ever heard. The story involves a man of mature age who had suffered from several psychological and medical problems most of his life. When the man was in his thirties, he was practically a cripple because of respiratory and circulatory problems. He also had a number of phobias — especially a fear of heights. He was advised against taxing himself and to live life as effortlessly as possible. He followed this advice for years but his condition didn't improve. He finally decided he was sick and tired of being sick and tired. While visiting a restaurant, he saw a picture of Mt. Blanc on the wall. He decided an excellent

way to overcome his fear of heights would be to climb Mt.
Blanc. He began telling his friends about his plans. He talked
about it so much to his friends that he had to do it. He began a
strenuous training program. He flew to Europe, hired a guide,
and actually climbed Mt. Blanc. Since then he has scaled it six
times. Hauck opines,

> Can you imagine the discipline it took for this middle-aged
> man to develop his body from that of a physical cripple to
> the point where he could actually keep up with experienced
> climbers? Can you imagine what it required for him to run
> several miles and swim many laps every day to prepare for
> this event? How many excuses would most of us come up
> with to escape this assignment? Yet despite the hardship,
> the difficulty, he has actually saved his life through this
> very program. In the final analysis, he was able to live in
> health for a long time, simply because he refused to evade
> the heavy responsibility of caring for his body.[1]

While this story is very impressive, there are many people
we know, whom we meet everyday, who exercise self-discipline.
There's the young wife who is an excellent mother, holds down
a job, and is a wonderful bed partner. She's climbing her moun-
tains at home.

There are many individuals who have inherited exquisite
genes but refuse to discipline themselves to do the things they
need to do to keep themselves in good health. By refusing to exercise the self-discipline required to take care of their bodies
they are actually inviting ailments, illnesses that could be
avoided. Conversely, there are others, who in spite of a predisposition to poor health, are willing to do the things they need to
do to promote good health. They value good health, are willing
to work for it, and in most cases succeed.

There are others who have the misfortune to inherit genes that predispose them to obesity and inertia. Suppose you are visiting a maternity ward and you look at the babies in the nursery. Do you see the baby who doesn't look alive, who isn't moving? You ask a nurse, "What's wrong with that baby?" "Nothing. It's just her nature," she replies.

That baby will probably grow into an adult who will ask others to bring things to her: "Please get me a glass of water. Please close the door. Please turn on the TV." She will take elevators, avoid movement of any kind. It's not her character, it's her nature. She is predisposed to avoid movement whenever possible.

The next baby is moving his hands and feet constantly. Something wrong here? No, just a genetic predisposition to activity. This baby will probably grow to be the adult who walks, runs, swims and has a jazzy metabolism — can eat almost anything he desires without gaining weight.

For people who are disinclined, who find it very difficult to exercise, that's the bad news. The good news is that these natural tendencies can be reversed. These very same people who by nature are predisposed to inactivity, can choose to avoid the physical ailments and illnesses that result from inactivity and poor eating habits. They can do for themselves what no doctor, no medication, no money can do for them. We're back to choices and making ourselves do the things we don't feel like doing.

Techniques of Self-Discipline

Like the idea of becoming a more disciplined person? Here are a few suggestions to get you started:

1. *Moderation.* Individuals who are overweight are usually compulsive personalities. All-or-Nothing people. They go

from abominable eating habits to diets where they become terrified when they have eaten two extra tablespoons of soup. The most important word in their vocabulary needs to be *moderation*. Try experimenting with foods you enjoy but exercise portion control. You will find you can have what you want if you're willing to restrict portions. Think about food like you think about your money. When you learn how much anything costs — a car, a friendship, a new dress — your awareness is sharpened. In this way you force yourself to put a value on what you want. Eat like slender people eat — REAL FOODS. Only fat people eat diet foods!

2. *Limit Your Goals.* Avoid "buying" into crash weight loss programs — avoid trying to lose a lot of weight quickly. "I must lose weight for the wedding." Even if the wedding is yours, it won't make that much difference, and you are again riding for a fall. The best way to change a lifestyle is to do it slowly. Gradual change is what healthy change is all about, but it does require focus and commitment. If making a lifestyle change is important to you, make it a priority, but limit the changes you can expect from yourself.

   Remember, it's OK to slip up now and then, but avoid having your slips add up. You do not want to feel guilty when you goof up because guilt could lead to overeating.

3. *Keep disciplined company.* It's amazing how much easier it is to break a bad habit if you have a buddy. Tell your friends that you're trying to lose weight and enlist their help and their interest. For example, have a party and prepare a tasty but healthy meal. Brag a little about your new interest in nutrition for yourself, your family, and your friends. Keeping disciplined company could be the breakthrough you've been searching for.

4. *Become a stoic.* Be willing to do tough tasks — having a mental attitude that says, no matter what, I can do it. With such an attitude, doing what you need to do will be less painful. Another way of saying the same thing is, doing hard things to get what you want is easier than the pain of not achieving your goal.

5. *Burn Your Bridges.* How often have you committed yourself to a task but retreated when the going got tough? But suppose you had no place to which you could retreat? Your only choice would be to become immobile or move forward. Stalin did this once when the Russians were in a battle with the Germans. He literally had the bridge burned so that the army had to stand its ground and fight for its very life. The Russians won, due in no small measure, many believe, to Stalin's strategy. It was either fight or die.

   Let's apply that same thinking to changing lifestyles. If Susie is willing to buy a dress for her daughter's wedding, pay more for it than she can afford, and deliberately select one size smaller than she can wear at the time of purchase, motivation will see her through. If at the same time she selects a way of eating she can live with, so much the better. The issue is *finding the motivation* to change a habit. Be brave. Burn your bridges by throwing out all the garbage foods in your house. Concentrate on keeping healthy foods and snacks around. If anyone in your house disagrees with your new eating style, apply the assertive techniques I describe in Chapter 4. Become a HEALTH NUT!

6. *Create a New Habit.* Make changes when you feel inspired. Go for it! There are many times when you have to push hard to make yourself do the things you don't feel like doing, but there are other times when you feel inspired, and you can't

wait to move, to do. This is the time to go for it! These times don't come that often, but when they do, *move*, be smart, and you'll accomplish tenfold during these periods. It's similar to being a salesman or a housewife. When you hit it hot as a salesman, refuse to stop with just a few sales. As they say, make hay while the sun shines. The same with housework. When you experience that rush of desire and energy to get it done, go for it. This is how some people get so much done. They capitalize on these moments of inspiration.

REBT Vocabulary:
How to Talk to Yourself in the Language of REBT

Every discipline has a language of its own. So here is a basic vocabulary of words and phrases that may serve as an introduction to the world of rational thinking. Learning this language can become a valuable and fascinating pursuit for you, just as it has for me.

During the early years of working with Living Thin I became obsessed with finding answers to why intelligent, thinking men, women and teenagers so often refuse to do the very things they needed to do to get what they wanted most — healthy and permanent weight control. I turned to my mentor who talked to me about the difficulty of changing habits of individuals who were not coping well with negative emotions that often caused the problem they were trying to overcome. All too often, they were using food as a tranquilizer, to soothe the "upsettedness"— eating in response to anger, anxiety, depression, boredom, and loneliness. Instead of resolving the emotional issues that bothered them, they used food as a temporary relief measure from these problems, thus winding up with three problems instead of one.

These people need to identify those negative emotions, label them, and then use their rational thinking skills to cope with them before going on to make lifestyle changes. The goal is simply to reduce and diffuse the intensity of your negative responses and at times even eliminate them, and whenever possible, to do it without the help of others so that thinking rationally becomes a habit that gives you the space to think clearly in any given situation.

It is important to understand that the purpose, the goal of learning and using this language is to help you think more clearly, more flexibly about your problems but not to do away with your emotional responses. Many people are fearful that by learning to become rational thinkers, they will begin thinking in robot-like fashion. Quite the contrary. Emotions are not irrational. Emotions that are appropriate are healthy. If you feel sorry, annoyed, regretful and disappointed when you fail to lose weight, that is rational when you have been doing your homework. This type of thinking in such a circumstance is good, healthy in fact. It's actually important that you do feel this way. I would hardly expect you to feel happy about failing to reach a goal when you have been working at resolving that problem.

Feeling inappropriately overwhelmed, "awfulizing," "horriblizing" about not losing weight, however, will lead only to failure. Exaggerating your feelings of disappointment will lead you, sooner or later, to unfortunate results and greater frustration. For example, I am disappointed that I am not losing weight as I think I should be, considering the effort I am investing, but

> **It's *never* Awful —**
> **just Inconvenient**
> **and Disappointing.**
> **You Can Stand it!**
> **You just Don't Like it.**

I refuse to give up, and I am determined to find answers. It's disappointing, but not horrible. It could be worse. I could be 75 pounds overweight rather than 45.

Let's begin by learning to identify basic emotions and familiarizing ourselves with some basic language.

Basic Emotions

Anger synonyms: annoyed, irritated, peeved, miffed, enraged, furious.

Pay attention to your language. The degree of emotion will be reflected in the words you choose to describe what you're feeling; i.e., feeling annoyed will produce feelings that are not nearly as intense as those described by the words "enraged" or "furious."

When I'm angry, there's a "should" in my head. I'm not getting the letter, the call, the recognition I *should* receive. The needle on the scale *should* be dropping more quickly. (Not getting what I want.)

Anxiety synonyms: fearful, terrified, scared, apprehensive.

A little bit of anxiety is healthy. If I'm standing on a busy corner — especially on a thoroughfare in New York City — I'd better be a little anxious about crossing the street. But if I allow that anxiety to reach a very high level — if it becomes excessive — I become immobilized. When I'm anxious, I'm suffering from what-if-itis. "*What if* I get on the plane and it crashes?"

My answer to that is, "As it goes down, you'll have time to worry. Why worry now? You may worry and worry, and it may not go down. So save your worry." Why go through life suffering from what-if-itis?

"*What if* I plan an outdoor wedding and it rains that day?"

Make your plans in advance, maybe have a backup plan, and take your chances. Just hope the marriage works.

"*What if* I give up the pie and I still fail to lose weight?"

At least you'll be healthier and you will have avoided gaining.

> Anger and Intolerance are the twin enemies of correct understanding.
>
> Mahatma Gandhi

Depression synonyms: sad, down, blue, dejected.

When I am depressed, I am feeling sorry for myself or others. Something happens and I say to myself, "Oh, I don't deserve that. That is so unfair. Poor me." The degree of depression is important too. Being sad or blue is not too worrisome, but if I become deeply depressed, that is a problem.

Guilt synonym: shame

When you are feeling guilty, you are beating on yourself and "shoulding" on yourself. "I *should* have done this. I *shouldn't* have done that." By eliminating these "shoulds," many feelings of guilt can be eliminated also.

Humiliation synonyms: shame, embarrassment, mortification.

I like the way Eleanor Roosevelt put it when she said, "No one can upset you without your consent." Likewise, no one can humiliate or embarrass you without your permission.

Frustration synonyms: impatience, annoyance.

Low frustration tolerance involves a belief that one cannot tolerate pain, discomfort, or adversity. The language associated with this emotion would be a) "I can't bear it"; b) "I can't live with (or without) it"; c) "I can't stand it"; and d) "I can't tolerate it." Can you understand why this kind of thinking can keep you upset most of the time?

It is important to understand that when talking about emotions, it's the degree or intensity of the feeling that determines whether the emotion is healthy or unhealthy. Sorrow, sadness, regret, frustration, anger, and annoyance are part of life for all of us. It would be unusual (inhuman, actually) not to feel this way from time to time. It's only when we allow the disappointment, sadness, anger or anxiety to overwhelm us and escalate into depression, rage, anxiety or panic that certain emotions become unhealthy and counterproductive.

In addition to emotions, there are several "stock" phrases that you need to understand in terms of REBT. I want you to begin thinking about what you're really saying when you use these expressions. For example, when you say, "I can't stand giving up sugar," or "I can't stand the way my mother-in-law talks to me," you don't really mean you can't stand it. What you really mean is, "I can stand giving up sugar; I can stand sitting down to dinner with my mother-in-law; I just don't like it."

When you say you can't stand something, it's as though having to go through the experience is lethal in its own right. Suppose you are lying on a table and your ankles and wrists are in chains. You cannot move. And very slowly and very deliberately a giant saw is coming toward you. When that saw reaches your body, it will slice you in half. And while the saw is coming you say, "I can't stand it, I can't stand it." But you are standing it. Until the saw actually slices you in half, you can stand it. You just don't like it, and you are fearful.

As this example illustrates, the language you choose to use has much to do with the way you feel and the way you think. Another way of saying this is, *The way I think, and the way I feel, and the way I behave are all interrelated, and the more awareness, the more information I have about how my thoughts create my feelings and behaviors, and how my behavior influences my thoughts and thinking, the more control, the more power I have. I find that I can actually even create the feeling I want to have by changing the thoughts in my head. It's very exciting!*

Another frequently heard and used "stinking-thinking" phrase is, "How dare she talk to me like that?" Several years ago a car dealership in Baltimore called me and suggested that I bring my car in to be serviced — there was something wrong. They asked me to arrive early, which I did. I came in, did some paperwork to bide the time, and when they were done, I got into my car and drove away. As I left, I noticed my tape deck wasn't working. I drove back immediately, called for the supervisor and explained the situation.

"My tape deck was working when I came in, but now that the car has been repaired, it's not working," I said.

He replied, "Mrs. Goldman, your tape deck was not working when you arrived this morning," to which I replied,

"You clearly did not hear me. It was working just before I drove my car into the service area."

"I don't think you understand," he continued. "I said it was not working when you arrived."

Getting angrier by the second, I countered, "What is your position here?"

"Assistant manager," he said.

"Is the manager here?" I demanded.

"Yes, upstairs."

"May I see him?"

"Of course," he replied.

I then told the entire story to the manager who basically told me his assistant manager was right and I was wrong. Although he repeated this message, I still found it difficult to comprehend. When I saw the assistant manager again he half-grinned and said, "What did he say?"

I replied, "You know very well what he said, but I am not leaving. I refuse. If you do not fix my tape deck, I will call my lawyer. I will not leave here otherwise. Is that clear?"

He then replied, "Fine. Johnny, please take care of Mrs. Goldman's car."

I retired to an office and did my work until he called.

"Here is your car, Mrs. Goldman," he said.

I got into my car feeling very superior, thinking I had handled a miserable situation very professionally, but upon reaching the street I discovered my tape deck still didn't work! I screamed, "How dare they? They asked me to come in. I never called them"!

I quickly realized, using my REBT skills, that if I allowed myself to continue becoming enraged and upset, I could easily have an accident or kill someone without ever knowing the *real* reason for my agitation, so I quickly changed my thoughts to "What can I do about it"?

I thought of an auto repair shop that specialized in repairing tape decks and felt better immediately. I also thought about reporting the managers to the owner of the dealership. The point is this: when you think of solutions, your anger is dissipated. You can't concentrate on both thoughts. By thinking of possible solutions you can calm yourself and get your thinking back on track. In other words, when you become very emotional, your rational thinking apparatus falters. The moment you begin to act rationally, your emotionality begins to diminish. It's diffused. A rational thinker will focus on solutions; an irrational thinker will begin "awfulizing" and "catastrophizing," which leads to escalating emotional responses and in some cases to overeating!

Another popular phrase is, "It's so unfair." Well, that's the way life is. Life is unfair. No one ever told you life was fair, not your parents, not your teachers, not your rabbis, not your priests. That's the way it is, and the sooner you accept it the less chance you have for becoming upset.

Another phrase we use in REBT is, "having a problem about having a problem." Often people get upset when they have problems. Rather than using their energy to resolve the problem, they're busy feeling sorry for themselves because they have a problem. That's called, "having a problem about having a problem." You now have two problems rather than one. Make sure you use your energy to find a solution to the problem instead of worrying about the problem.

Another aspect of learning REBT is understanding the difference between *needs* and *wants*. When I'm in an airplane and the plane begins falling and an oxygen mask drops down in front of me, it's more than wanting the oxygen mask; I need that oxygen to survive. *It's more than want.* But when I say I *need* to lose weight, unless I am very sick, it's not a need; I *want* to lose weight.

> **The Essence of REBT can be summed up in three words. Can you Guess? TOUGH — TOO BAD!**

Saying I *need* it and *want* it are two different things. Strive to recognize the difference between needs and wants. A need is something you absolutely cannot do without. A want is something you'd like to have, but it's not a must.

Coping Statements For Specific Situations

Situation: "I'm not accustomed to exercising. It's too hard to incorporate even 3–5 minutes of exercise into my day."
Response: "It's never too hard, it's just hard, and if you refuse to do even 3–5 minutes, your problem will increase. So will your waistline."

Situation: "Now that I'm eating healthily I have to cook two meals instead of one because my husband insists on sticking with his slovenly eating habits. It's so unfair."
Response: "So it's unfair. Did anybody ever tell you life was fair?"

Situation: "I've been working on making changes and have lost only four pounds in four weeks. I don't think it's working."
Response: "Then I'll just have to work a little harder, but I refuse to give up."

Situation: "When I go to a party, I need to eat the pastries and goodies I'm accustomed to eating."
Response: "You don't *need* what you want. You may want it, but you don't need it."

> Learn how to live with neurotic people.
> People have a right to be depressed.
> People have a right to be angry.
> People have a right to be neurotic.
> Everybody has RIGHTS!

Above all, always remember: YOU DON'T HAVE TO FEEL LIKE DOING IT. YOU JUST HAVE TO DO IT.

Can you now understand how the language, the words, the phrases you choose to use will create feelings both positive and negative? Let's get rid of the "shoulds," the "musts," the "oughts" and exchange them for preferences and desires. And remember, the only person you can control is yourself.

It's important to remember that everyone has Rights! Uncle Harry has a right to have as many wives as he can afford (but hopefully not at the same time). His daughters also have the right to hate him for it, to begrudge the money he is spending on other women. Everyone has Rights! Granting people the right to have rights will make it easier for you to lose weight. How? What's the connection? Because you'll be letting go of emotional upsets that cause you to nibble and nosh. By giving up your "shoulds" and accepting the rights of others, you are freeing yourself of negative emotions that make change impossible.

There is no one way to lose weight. By watching your language you will begin making clearer and more rational choices about your eating habits.

New ABCs of Rational Thinking:
A Formula To Rid Yourself of "Stinking Thinking"

Here is a systematic method — a formula for talking to yourself when you are feeling negative emotions.

Let's say I am feeling low. What is the problem? In spite of many friends and interests, I am alone. When I return from a trip, there is no one to rejoice with me other than "friends" who may not be there when you want them.

First, let's identify the problem and accept the fact that my feelings are not coming from the reasons I've just cited. They are coming from my thoughts, my words — phrases I'm choosing to tell myself. These words and thoughts happen automatically. I am not even aware of my choice of words.

Our goal in teaching you to think more rationally is to help you understand that the way you think is often a collection of thinking habits you've picked up along the way, and these habits are causing you to feel as you do. That's the bad news. But the good

> Remember, it's not the hurdles in the road that cause you to be upset, it's the way you handle the hurdles.
>
> **The Hurdles Are the Road!**

news is these thinking patterns can be changed; and what is more uplifting than change? It's the stuff of good health, similar to opening a window and letting in some fresh air.

Here is a formula for thinking rationally:

A. The event: I just returned from a trip. I had a glorious time, but as I said, there is no one around to greet me other than friends — no significant other. In fact, my choice of a significant other just selected a dear friend of mine to be his significant other.

B. Head talk: I'll never find another Harry. He's one in a million. I can't bear the thought of compromising and accepting someone with whom I have no "chemistry."

C. Feelings: down, sad, depressed.

At issue here is that my feelings do NOT come from the event, although you may find that difficult to believe. They come from the "B"— my head talk. Just suppose I changed my B (head talk) to, "Boy, am I glad I don't have to answer to anyone when I return from a trip," or "How lucky I am to be free of annoying or undesirable entanglements! I can do

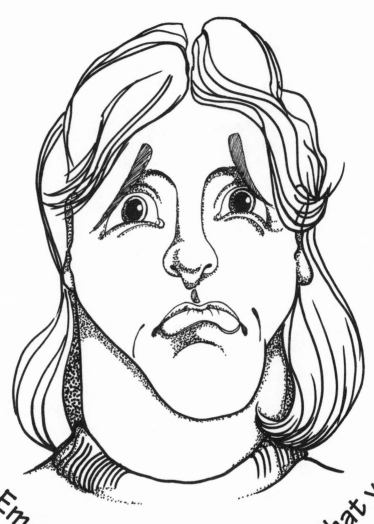

Emotional pain comes from what you say in your head about a situation — "He doesn't love me anymore — I can't stand it"

whatever turns me on." If I say it long enough, I will begin believing it. Identify your head talk.

D. Dispute, challenge head talk

Now's the time to dispute, challenge my head talk, but first I need to identify it. I need to pinpoint my head talk. I need to be a detective, to ask myself, "What am I saying" and stay focused. I'm saying:

1. *I'll never find another Harry.*

   Never? How can I prove that? I might find someone today, this afternoon. I better keep myself feeling up. If I am busy and meeting people, one never knows. NEVER is a meaningless word!

2. *I can't bear the thought . . . I CAN'T BEAR THE THOUGHT!*

   I can stand it, and someday I may take Robert if I can't have Harry.

   By questioning and challenging these thoughts I begin feeling better. I begin realizing that I was exaggerating the situation. Does it erase the problem? No, but it does diffuse it, reduce the intensity, and as a result, I feel better, lighter about the situation.

E. Choices: This is the best part of the formula. I have choices!

1. I can make plans to meet more people. This activity will remove the sting of the loneliness that I dislike. In fact, it will give me something to look forward to. How fortunate that I am alone.

2. I can also begin to create situations that will increase my chances for meeting people. I think I'll make a list.

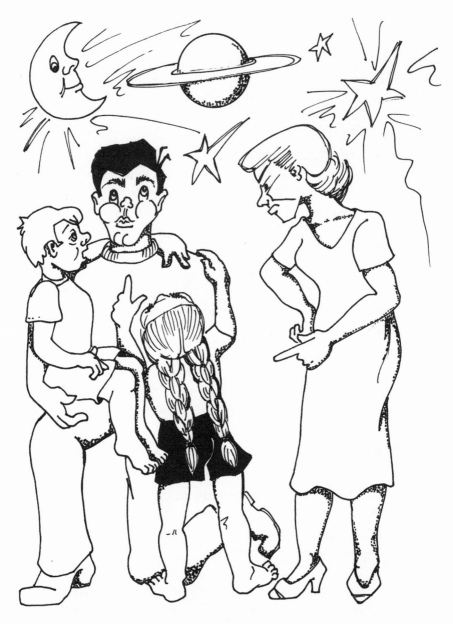

I refuse to SHOULD on myself,
my friends, my family,
or the universe!

3. I can also refuse to do anything — just wail and whine about the situation — an excellent way to increase my depression.*

Rational Thinking For Living Thin

1. *Irrational*: I am helpless to control my urge to eat food and cannot be held accountable for what I put in my mouth.

   Rational: I have enormous control over what I choose to put in my mouth.

2. *Irrational*: Because I am overweight, I know everyone finds me unattractive and repulsive.

   Rational: While there may be many advantages to being slender and looking attractive to others, I don't need the approval of others to feel good about myself.

3. *Irrational*: It is easier to avoid such things as reducing the amount of food I eat than to face self-responsibility for controlling my intake and focusing on personal growth.

   Rational: What may appear to be an easy way will invariably be much harder and more painful in the long run.

4. *Irrational*: I've lost a few pounds, and *I must not gain them back*, no matter what, or I will be defeated and forced to give up.

   Rational: Change is tough and takes time. Just because I occasionally goof does not mean I'm a failure. That's ridiculous.

---

* **Important:** For many people, learning the basics of rational thinking will help them become better problem solvers and to indeed learn how to talk to themselves. But if your problem is intense or you can't help yourself, don't hesitate to see a qualified REBT therapist. To locate an REBT therapist in your area, contact the Albert Ellis Institute, 45 East 65th Street, New York, NY 10021-6593. Phone: (212) 535-0822; Fax: (212) 249-3582.

THINK STRAIGHT INSTEAD OF CROOKED!

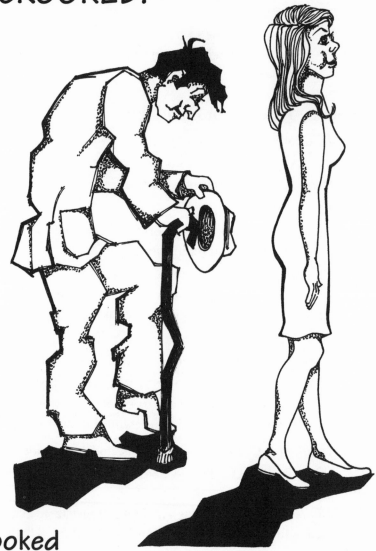

Crooked thinking

He should

I should

They should

QUESTION: WHY?

Straight thinking

Why shouldn't they?

5. *Irrational*: Because I've
   been overweight for some
   time, that proves I need
   someone to help me gain
   control of my weight
   problem, someone other
   than myself on whom to
   rely.

> You take yourself
> with you wherever
> you go.
>
> Emerson

Rational: Depending on others is a big part of my problem.
I'd better begin thinking and acting independently.

6. *Irrational*: I am overweight for a host of complex reasons,
   and only a highly educated and intelligent person can understand my problems.

   Rational: The problem is simple! Weight loss is scientific.
   When I eat more calories than my body requires to maintain
   my present weight, I will gain weight.

7. *Irrational*: My emotional cravings for food are often intoler-
   able and must be controlled by eating.

   Rational: Some discomfort is a necessary, inevitable and entirely harmless part of losing weight. At these times I'll be
   willing to satisfy my cravings with low-calorie, healthy foods
   like carrots, apples, and other veggies.

Self-Confidence

Self-confidence, or self-efficacy, comes from a firm belief I
can overcome obstacles. I can assume responsibility for myself.
I don't need others to tell me what to eat or do. Self-confidence
comes from believing I can assume responsibility for myself; I
am not a wimp; I refuse to live as a victim; I can make my own

decisions; I don't have to be perfect; and I can learn to Live Thin if I choose.

Self-respect is something I earn for myself when I do hard things. No one can give it to me. I won't increase my self-esteem by having someone tell me how handsome or good looking I am, or by having someone tell me how wonderful I am. No one can give me self-esteem as though it were a gift. It's not for sale.

Conclusion

REBT is all about growing up. Ellis tells us that people get older but they refuse to grow up. They remain children in many respects. Lillian Hellman says it another way in her play *Toys in the Attic*; the characters get older but they still insist on playing with the toys in the attic. They still cling to childish modes of thought and behavior.

We assume that mature people make decisions that are logical and rational. But when even mature individuals allow their emotions to overwhelm them, they can easily lose control of their reasoning powers and become victimized by their excessive emotional reactions.

The good life is really about maturity. The person who is mature, who is willing to hang in, who refuses to give up, has what it takes to be a good problem solver.

As a society we've been deceived into believing that the "good life" embraces a lifestyle that is free of all responsibility, and that retirement is the goal of a happy life. The converse is true! A life without change, without challenge can be pretty dull. If being overweight has been a problem, you now have a blueprint for success that gives you two-for-one: more health and less stress. You have the basics. You have the ammunition. Remember you'll be using your REBT for the rest of the book. Without mastering the basics of sound mental health your chances of winning your battle with weight control will indeed be slender!

Why was REBT included and why did it become the most important part of my Living Thin Program? Early on, it became painfully clear that the students in my classes were unwilling to do the things they needed to do to take weight off and keep it off, healthily and permanently. Their problems were usually psychological. The individual who is not coping with daily stress is not ready for change: e.g., "Don't ask me to give up my addiction when I am depressed, anxious, angry, bored, or lonely. It's not only *hard* but *TOO HARD*."

The key to change is motivation. If the pleasure of eating the hot fudge sundae is greater than the pleasure of watching the needle on the scale drop, the sundae will win. But here is the good news: motivation waxes and wanes, and as you learn more about motivation, and as you learn to think and talk more rationally, it will become easier for you to do what it takes to hold onto it. Giving up garbage food will be easier. The first garbage you want to give up is the GARBAGE IN YOUR HEAD!

You can retrain your head. Is it easy to start a new habit? No. Is it worthwhile? You decide. Think of the consequences of not doing it vs. doing it.

Rational thinking is "generalizable." By that I mean you can use it to help you think rationally about lots of things. You use it all day long if you are emotionally healthy. Each time you think rationally, it means you are doing your homework or that you think rationally without even thinking about how you are thinking. Some individuals — not many — are born with a talent for rational thinking.

The single most important part of an individual is the way that individual feels about him- or herself. If you have goals, go for them, and work for them. Force yourself; you'll love the results. Always remember, you don't have to feel like doing it. You just have to do it.

I know you are "champing at the bit" to get started. But trust me when I tell you that you are not ready for the journey. There is work to be done before you can think about losing weight.

The purpose of my Living Thin Program is making sure that you are not being victimized by your emotions. Taking on the responsibility of changing your eating habits is a laborious task. To keep your motivation in shape you need all your mental "muscle" in top form. You can't be the captain of your own ship when you are overreacting to daily stress, which in turns leads in many cases to eating problems. In other words, without this emotional control your goose will be cooked! So forget the magic bullets. Remember, those magic bullets never work, and the long cut is actually the short cut. So for a shortcut that works, read on.

3

Step Into My Classroom
and Let's Get Started

"I Know What To Do, So Why Don't I Do It?"

You say you know what to do to lose weight. So why don't you do it?

I'll tell you why. You don't do it because you don't feel like doing it. That's the problem, plain and simple. And the problem's solution is always the same: **YOU DON'T HAVE TO FEEL LIKE DOING IT, YOU JUST HAVE TO DO IT!** You'll feel like doing it later.

Before this chapter ends, you will begin your Living Thin journey, but first we need to attack and challenge the GARBAGE IN YOUR HEAD. The garbage is simply a reflection of attitudes you have on specific issues that stops you from getting started. The solution is freeing yourself from the garbage by learning to think RATIONALLY. If you choose to ignore the garbage in your head — to allow it to reside there as always — you will need to think about the consequences: obesity, poor health, diminished self-esteem, annoyance, frustration, self-loathing, anxiety, and, very likely, a lifetime of unsuccessful dieting.

You may say,

- *I simply do not have the time to study all the information on healthy weight loss and good eating*
- *I am too busy and too tired to have to think about it*
- *My motivation never lasts*
- *There are so many articles and so many books, so many programs — It's confusing*
- *Besides, what's wrong with wanting fast and easy weight loss?*

Sounds great, that last one, but it just doesn't work! That's what's wrong with it. Everyone talks about the issue of TIME. Then why devote time, effort, and dollars to programs that are destined to fail? If diet programs succeeded, the sponsoring companies would soon be out of business. Failure is a built-in component. They depend on it! The answer is to educate yourself, to be in charge. And being in charge is exactly what you are on the verge of doing.

Let's not overlook another problem — insisting on easy answers. This problem often leads to allowing yourself to be exploited by people, all too willing to sell you potions and pills, especially antiobesity pills. Those desperate for easy answers say, "If it gets to where I have no other choice, I can always take the antiobesity pills. Surely, there is no harm in them. After all, doctors prescribe them." Well, I have news for you. Not only do they not work, they can cause serious illness.

David Levitsky, professor of nutritional sciences and psychology at Cornell University and a nationally known expert on the control of obesity, reported in the January/February 1997 issue of *Healthy Weight Journal* that Redux (a brand name for d-fenfluramine, the most popular antiobesity pill at the time) is associated with sleep problems, headaches, dizziness, nervousness, anxiety, depression, and abnormal dreams, and that discontinuing the drug is related to depression, delusion, hypertension, and nausea.

Anything artificial can't be healthy. And equally as important, when you depend on a pill, you are not changing your eating and thinking habits. Therefore, the consequence is that after you have lost some weight you return to your old habits and repeat the cycle.

Past experience with losing and gaining weight does make a difference. After questioning and working with several thousand people over the course of many years and doing my own research, I have learned that "dieting" unquestionably slows the metabolism. If I question a group of twenty women about their past weight loss efforts, the answers range from, "I can't lose weight eating approximately 1800 calories," to, "I can't lose weight on approximately 1100 calories." While the reasons are mixed, the women who cannot lose weight on 1800 calories have clearly never dieted, while the ones who can't lose on approximately 1100 calories have dieted rigorously for a long period. The solution for the slow loser is more exercise, whenever possible, and gradual but deliberate and radical change in eating habits. Listening to men and women discuss their failed "solutions" for losing weight convinces me that easy answers are destined to fail.

Now that we've identified what doesn't work, let's turn our attention to what does. What works is education on every level, from what happens when you spend too many calories on nutritionally empty food, to how you manage stress and how to fix attitudes. If you refuse to educate yourself and make your own decisions, you are at the mercy of every huckster who comes along. Only an educated person can accept the fact that gradual change is the best method for accomplishing permanent change.

To make the necessary changes to meet your goal, you need to change the underlying conditions that have given rise to your problem. You need to understand the reasons for indulging in certain eating patterns and lifestyle choices, because these are the habits that have created the problem in the first place.

There's nothing magic about losing weight. A lot of people know how to do it. The problem is, it's not a diet that's going to do it. It's a change in lifestyle.

What bothers me about all the systems that are now being marketed nationwide for millions if not billions of dollars is that they're not honest. They promise you something that they can only deliver in the short term . . . .

The only way that [people] can really maintain any kind of a good habit is to learn techniques that will help them to design a program in which they can help themselves.[1]

David Hungerford, M.D.

Additionally, you need to understand that diets, whether you are running your own or are participating in a program, are costly. They are expensive in terms of what happens to your body as you lose and gain, in terms of losing confidence in yourself and continuing poor nutritional habits, and also in how these poor habits affect you as you age.

The creators of diet programs do not want you to realize that your failure to achieve permanent success is structured into the program. When you accept a weight loss program that fails you, all you are learning to do is to be dependent on the program. And you might consider that if your eating habits are based on what someone else says you should eat, you are on someone else's diet, not yours. Diet programs that are designed for "everyone" are, in fact, for no one. For new dietary patterns to work, they need to be based on your lifestyle and personal preferences. The decisions you make to lose weight or gain health do not have to be perfect, but they do have to be your own.

Eating Chart, "Suggested" Meal Plans — Aids to Get Started

At the end of Chapter 5 I have included some meal plan suggestions for Living Thin. Don't panic. They are not rigid meal plans you must follow. Living Thin is not a diet! I only include them as examples of nutritious, low-calorie meals. Feel free to use your own ideas as well as mine. You must devise meals that work for you. You must be in charge of you. These menus are merely a way of getting you started on your Living Thin and Living Young journey.

I have also included an eating chart on the following page. This is one of the most useful tools for losing weight you will ever find. During the course of a week write down everything

The Write Way to Learn: People who succeed in losing weight and keeping it off keep food diaries. Those who fail don't.

Days	Breakfast	Cal.	Lunch	Cal.	Dinner	Cal.	Snacks	Cal.	Tot. Cal.	Water	Exercise
Monday											
Tuesday											
Wednesday											
Thursday											
Friday											
Saturday											
Sunday											

you eat and when you eat it. The purpose of your chart is to help you develop an awareness of what and why you choose to eat. Your goal is to find a way of eating that will be enjoyable, a way of eating that means you are never hungry, and you are making choices that will make your body happy and healthy.

Avoid thinking of calories at this point. In fact, in your next chapter I will give you two approaches, one with calories, one without. You will make the choice.

ASSIGNMENT 1

For your first assignment in getting started, simply force yourself to write down everything you eat without counting calories. The eating chart is the least expensive and best ally you will ever have. It helps you to learn about your most favorite person, you. View it as a challenge, not a chore. I promise you the minute you begin doing this, you'll be on your way to gaining control of your eating habits.

At this point we're ready to examine and attack the garbage in your head that stops you from GETTING STARTED. The garbage is simply a by-product of the attitudes you harbor about a variety of issues. What does your attitude have to do with losing weight? Everything! Food is only 10 percent of the problem. Attitude is the other 90 percent.

An attitude is what we CHOOSE to tell ourselves about any given subject — in this case, weight loss. Our attitudes cause us to think the way we think.

> **TAKE CHARGE OF YOUR ATTITUDE. Don't Let Someone Else Choose It For You.**

The way we think is connected to the way we feel about ourselves. The way we feel about ourselves is connected to the way we behave.

That means you have enormous power — enormous control over your behavior. Your attitude reflects your beliefs. Your beliefs, in turn, are based on your experiences.

You are not married to these beliefs, however. You don't have to cling to them. Sound mental health means you understand that if your behavior is self-defeating, it is getting in the way of achieving your goals, in this case, a healthy weight loss. You can't change your height or the color of your eyes, but you can change your attitude. It's similar to spring house cleaning. You throw open the drapes and get the dust bunnies out of the crevasses of your mind — you open the windows and let the air carry your stale ideas away. In other words, you air out your brain and replace your "stinking thinking" with fresh, wholesome thinking.

> **What we think about, we move toward or we move away from. Our thoughts largely or partly, not completely, control our feelings.**

On to "Stinking Thinking" — Dealing with Denial

Telling the truth is the first step. You will never get what you want if you are having difficulty admitting that you have a problem. Not admitting you have a problem means that you are having a problem about "having a problem." You need to be willing to accept that there is a problem to start with, and then move on to discover what the problem is specifically. The success of Alcoholics Anonymous is based on the members admitting that they have a real problem.

We all have habits, urges, and thought patterns that interfere with our moving ahead and reaching goals. Here are three ways for coping with our problems.

A. DENY IT. Pretend it doesn't exist. Lie about it. Turn your head the other way. Buy a dress size several sizes smaller than you need and have your dressmaker add extra material to make it larger so you can wear it. Then tell others that they can see by the label that it is a size 12, even though you and they know that a size 20 would have been a better fit.

B. FIND ANOTHER DIET. Try diet after diet. Refuse to assume responsibility for yourself. Wail and whine when you continue to lose and gain.

C. ADMIT THE PROBLEM. VIEW IT AS AN ADVENTURE IN LEARNING. SEE IT AS A CHALLENGE. This is the ideal solution. Refuse to become upset, and when you find an intelligent, common sense approach, experiment with it until you find a solution that works for you. Learn about SELF-TALK. (See end of this chapter.) Practice statements such as, "It's not too hard, it's just hard . . . and so what," and "I am determined to be in charge . . . No more diets . . . DIETS ARE FOR DUMMIES." However, I need to be ready to change for the right reasons — not because my doctor thinks I need it or my mother-in-law thinks I am too fat. If my behavior fails to match my so-stated goals, that tells me I am not ready, and that's OK. I am

> **Make Failure A New Beginning.**

not a failure because I am not ready. I am perhaps just Not
Ready. Accepting the problem will make it easier to move
through the problem instead of around it.

Attitudes About Health and Nutrition

I am reminded of a scene from the play *The Man Who Came
To Dinner* whenever I encounter the following attitude about
health and nutrition. Sadly, it is more prevalent today than I care
to admit.

In one scene a nurse tells her patient, Monte Wooley, whose
character is very ill, lying in a hospital bed, "You are to have no
candy while you are ill." His reply? "My mother ate a box of
chocolates every day of her life. She lived to be 103 and when
she was dead for three days, she looked better than you do now."

So often I have heard about someone who knows someone
who lived to a very advanced age while eating gobs of refined
sugar, grease, etc., but can we guarantee that you will live forever, free of illness if you are nutritionally correct all the time?
Of course not! There are no such guarantees. But if our health
scientists have learned anything about our bodies and the importance of nutrition, you might be interested to learn a little on the
subject.

You can raise the probability of better health by eating
healthily. Your body knows the difference between health and illness and, without your good decision making, will express those
differences all too clearly for some of you. Here are some powerful, sobering, and instructive thoughts from the internationally
respected, best selling author David Reuben, M.D.

> You have been tricked into liking a breakfast of artificial-
> imitation-synthetic orange drink, imitation white bread,

imitation butter (margarine), imitation jam (made with corn syrup), chemicalized coffee with imitation cream and possibly imitation eggs and imitation bacon. You gulp artificial-imitation-synthetic vitamin and mineral pills covered with artificial colors. You eat 5000 different synthetic chemicals in your day-to-day diet, and you consume more than six pounds of exotic preservatives and artificial chemical compounds every year. You suffer from an epidemic of obesity, heart attacks, diabetes and cancer unheard of in the history of the world — most of which comes from your rotten diet. The gigantic food processors and food sellers spend more than two billion dollars a year to tell you how well you are eating and how nutritious your awful artificial-chemical-laden diet is.

Penny for penny and pound for pound, you eat one of the worst diets in the world — and it is hurting you and your children more than you are willing to admit. Slide your hands down over your stomach and see how much fat you carry there. Run your tongue over your teeth and check the number of cavities your imitation diet has brought you. Think of your friends and relatives with cancer, diabetes and heart attacks — and think of the rotten food they ate to get that way.[2]

Dr. Reuben is telling the men and women of America that the greatest risk to their well-being is not nuclear bombs but what's on their plate at mealtime. And I am telling you that weight loss is 10 percent food and 90 percent attitude. The

> It's no longer a question of staying healthy. It's a question of finding a sickness you like.
>
> Jackie Mason

solution to this problem is to be WILLING to change your attitude about nutrition and health.

Dealing With Low Frustration Tolerance

Let me illustrate low frustration tolerance. You want what you want immediately or, at least, overnight. In your head is the message, *"I need to have a program that is not only easy and works immediately but one that I don't even have to think about."*

This type of thinking and this desire feed the weight loss industry to the tune of approximately $4 billion a year. The weight loss industry continues to make huge profits thanks to your and other DC's huge failure to understand low frustration tolerance. That same failure keeps you glued to programs that promise quick results "without any hassles," but which ultimately guarantee your failure to lose weight permanently.

LFT means you have a low tolerance for frustration — not only for losing weight but daily living. Too many "shoulds" keep you feeling upset too much of the time. Example: *"I can't stand to wait in line to see a movie,"* or *"I can't bear slow traffic."*

When working on this portion of the book, I went to the pharmacy. As I waited to give my order, I met a gal I hadn't seen for several years. She told me how frustrated she was about the traffic where we both live and that in spite of the area being beautifully planned and a "privileged" place to live, she simply, "could not stand it" and was planning to move for that reason. Unwilling to put

> The problem of life is not to make life easier, but to make men stronger.
>
> H. A. Montague

up with traffic, she also refused to acknowledge that traffic in her new community may very soon be busier than where she lives now.

While I noticed her anger I also noted that she had gained a good hunk of weight (could tell by her double chin, bloated look, and protruding tummy). Now let's explore how her impatience can "extend" to her stomach.

Since we live in a very crowded and complicated society, a low tolerance for frustration will result in your walking around angry and upset much of the time. In other words, you want immediate gratification and find any type of discomfort entirely unacceptable, which can lead to candy bars and chocolate cake for comfort.

If you derive pleasure from something that has harmful side effects, i.e., high calorie junk foods and other high-calorie, empty-value foods, you clearly will not enjoy that pleasure very long. Yes, you will experience considerable pleasure in the short term, but more pain than pleasure in the long run. When you insist on resisting doing what you need to do to get what you want, you are saying, *"I shouldn't have to do anything that is unpleasant or uncomfortable. And I'd sooner maintain the status quo than risk discomfort."* While you clearly have a right to live by such a philosophy, it will surely lead to unhappiness by blocking you from reaching your goals. Your head talk goes something like, *"I can't bear it. I can't live with (or without) it. It's too hard. I can't stand it. I can't tolerate it,"* etc.

Recognizing and taking responsibility for self-control is the ultimate in being liberated.

What's the best defense against such thinking? Practice saying, *It's never TOO hard, it's just hard — or I CAN stand it, I just don't like it.*

Here's another example. I recall vividly working with a young man in his thirties who talked incessantly about his feelings of intense deprivation when others were enjoying rich desserts. The mere thought of having to have fruit rather than the rich desserts he adored infuriated him. Unless, and until, "Sam" is willing to change his own self-talk, his chances for slimming down are null and void. He needs to be willing to let go of his childish talk before he can even think about wearing the handsome jackets he purchases, always hoping they will fit one day.

LFT is the single most important and most obvious problem for people trying to change their habits. LFT differs from plain ordinary frustration. While ordinary frustration means being troubled or upset by how things are, LFT is actually a form of laziness and resentment. It is expressed as a refusal to do what needs to be done. This is the number one reason many people find change painfully difficult — not just changing habits in order to lose weight, although that's what we are dealing with here.

LFT is responsible for the following negative thinking patterns that interfere with change:

1. WAMPING YOURSELF — Saying things like, *"I'll never make it. I try and always fall backward, which proves I am destined to always fail."*

    This statement needs to be changed to, "So I slipped, I'm not perfect. So what? If others can make it, so can I. I refuse to give up. No matter how often I fail, I will pick myself up and try again."

2. CAN'T STAND IT-ITIS — Thinking you "can't stand" giving up sweets, especially when you are with people eating

sweets right in front of you. In other words, the pleasure of the moment is more important to you than the pleasure of reaching a goal. Immediate gratification wins out over long-term objectives.

However, I am telling you that overcoming the pleasure of the immediate moment requires planning and practice. This "planning" and "practice" is called DISCIPLINE. Like all habits, it becomes stronger with repetition. The payoff is achieving your goal, increased self-esteem, and becoming a role model for yourself and others.

Here are the statements that "losers" use to enhance their LFT:

- *"It's not only hard to change, it's too hard and it shouldn't be that hard"*
- *"It's awful that I have to count calories to win my weight battle"*
- *"I simply can't tolerate planning and having to think about changing my eating and activity patterns, even though I know I am doing it for my health — both mental and physical"*

Remember to tell yourself, "It's never too hard to change, it's just hard. And so what?" It's not awful to count calories, it's just annoying until you become accustomed to it.

What you need to do is pinpoint the statements you use in your head that "feed" your LFT, and challenge those statements! You will learn to be your own best friend (and therapist) by beginning to dispute these thoughts and accept that there is no gain without pain. No matter how hard you find change to be, you will inevitably find that not changing is even harder as you go through life becoming increasingly more dissatisfied. Plus, you know that the longer you wait the harder it gets.

> Most tough decisions are simple.
> It's just tough living them out.

By using the skills I am helping you develop you will, in time, overcome your resistance. As you experience the pleasure of the improvements, your motivation to continue will increase as well.

Here are a few scenarios that LFT leads to:

TWO-YEAR-OLD-ISM — You insist that you get what you want on your own terms — perhaps to keep eating sweets. What are your terms? They are to keep eating sweets but maybe give them up a little, but not completely. To do a little exercise, but not much. Not to have to keep an eating chart and not having to plan. In other words, you want to lose weight easily, painlessly, without hassles and without having to "think about it."

To overcome this kind of "guaranteed-to-make-you-fail thinking" you need to be willing to get tough with yourself. You begin doing, not just talking about doing, hard things like changing your head talk.

When your head talk is saying, "It's too hard," you challenge that by saying, "No, it's just hard, not too hard. I am not going to react like a two-year-old. I'm not a two-year-old any longer who demands that life gives me what I want on my terms." Letting the former head talk get by is like watering your LFT plant. By making yourself do uncomfortable things, you will eventually find it fairly easy to do the very things you now find hard to do.

If your head talk says you can't stand the idea of keeping an eating chart or doing a little exercise because it's too awful, remember, you will respect yourself in the morning if you can dispute and challenge those exaggerated statements in your head.

All the things you say may be a little true; yes, it's inconvenient and perhaps not preferable, but don't exaggerate by saying it's awful or unbearable.

The last thing to be said about solutions for overcoming your LFT is this: Talking won't help and complaining won't help. What works is doing something about it.

The Pitfalls of Grandiosity — Little-King Syndrome

Often another obstacle to change is grandiosity, or what I call the Little-King Syndrome. Grandiosity, an infrequently used term, is often misunderstood. Simply put, grandiosity describes the actions of people who believe they do not have to play by the conventional rules that apply to everyone else. These grandiose people believe that there are special rules just for them.

You have already heard about Sherri whose idea of having fun was eating nachos and drinking beer at ball games. She failed to understand the scientific nature of weight loss and looked for miracles. None was available for her nor for Elizabeth Taylor either. You remember I saw Sherri some time later at a food fair. She looked great, and told me she finally got the message.

Confronting Boredom and Loneliness

"When I'm feeling bored, lonely, I turn to food, and while I am thinking about food and while I am nibbling and noshing, I'm no longer bored or lonely." I hear that often in my classes. That's the good news. The bad news is she now has two problems instead of one. She's still feeling bored and lonely, but now she has probably gained another pound!

The solution for coping with your boredom and loneliness is the very same solution I'm suggesting for all your problems.

Grow up! Assume responsibility for yourself. Avoid waiting for others to cure your boredom and loneliness.

The problem of boredom and loneliness is actually created when we allow ourselves to become passive spectators instead of active participants. There is scientific data that tells us that a willingness to remain passive has been proven to be psychologically self-destructive and is actually a chronic illness.

Get involved. Make a list of your interests. Force yourself to work at finding a niche that will work for you. When you are busy helping others, you simply don't have the time to be bored and lonely. The key lies in forcing yourself to do the things you don't feel like doing. **You don't have to FEEL like doing it, you just have to DO IT if you want to get rid of your boredom and loneliness.** Think of the consequences of allowing yourself to feel bored or depressed. Your motivation will be eroded — destroyed. And when you lose your motivation, change is impossible.

Motivation and Change

> *"If you insist on doing what you've always done, you'll always get what you've always gotten."*

In spite of this wisdom, many people — especially you — resist change because change is tough. Motivation is the key that will give you what you want. It will open the door for you. The issue is, where can you go to find this motivation? It is natural to want, even yearn, for someone to do it for you, to motivate you to do the things you want to do. During my many years of teaching the Living Thin classes, I frequently heard the following explanation for failure, "Sure, if I were more like Mary, I could lose weight. She has the self-discipline, the willpower that I simply lack." I've heard the same story, different names, more times than I care to remember.

On the other hand, I've also heard another story frequently. My students would report that after a class they would talk about Living Thin to their friends with great excitement, and when the friend would ask, "What exactly was Sylvia talking about?" they were at a loss to say exactly what the class was about. Having attended the class thirty minutes earlier, they couldn't remember what had been said.

Why was this, you ask? Because what they were excited about and what their friends so easily recognized, was that they were feeling stimulated, optimistic, eager — in other words, MOTIVATED. All I did was strike the match and they were on fire with their own motivation. Now you are saying, "Well, someone else struck the match for them." You're right, I did. But what they learned in class and what I am teaching you is TO LIGHT YOUR OWN MATCH! Many people wish that someone or something would come along and supply the motivation.

Motivation is like any other subject. The more you know about it, the more control you have. A new driver behind the wheel of a car is confused about what to do first, what is safe, and what those pedals are for. Being uneducated about motivation leads to the same paralysis and confusion.

The single most effective tool for motivating yourself to do what you really want to do is to force yourself to take action . . . whether you feel like it or not. The desire to continue will be your reward. I promise.

Motivation: How It Works and How to Manage It
So It Will Work For You

"When I am highly motivated, I can do hard things, but when I lose my motivation, I find it impossible to do the things I need to do." Sound like anyone you know?

Motivation has a life of its own. It is natural for your motivation to come and go. It's here . . . then it's gone. It waxes and wanes. What motivates you today may not motivate you tomorrow. That's OK because you know it will return — providing you refuse to give up, providing you are willing to do hard things first, and providing you force yourself to take some action. Motivation will then follow. Too many people sit around waiting for the motivation they need to bestir themselves. Motivation comes to those who are willing to force themselves to do hard things. However, you need to want your goal enough to be willing to make yourself do hard things. (We come back again to the issue of how much do you want it? Are you willing to do the things you need to do?)

On Tuesday you may find that your desire for a hot fudge sundae is stronger than your desire to lose a pound. On Tuesday you will lose that battle. Accept it. Go with it. Enjoy your sundae. However, on Wednesday you may find that your desire to lose some weight is far greater than your desire to indulge in a dessert. On that day your desire to lose weight will win over the dessert. Whichever feeling is stronger will win.

Be on guard and refuse to "wamp" yourself if you relapse. Similarly, if your desire to achieve perfection is stronger than your desire to experiment with intelligent, rational approaches for weight loss, you may find yourself giving up before you even begin. A perfectionist very often would rather give up than accept the imperfection of winning on Monday and losing on Tuesday. So avoid the need for being perfect.

Motivation is a complicated and fascinating issue. Let's untangle the mystery by studying the following examples.

1. Marilyn — a stunning, well-dressed woman and mother of two, tells me she is determined to win the Living Thin game. But she becomes increasingly depressed and angry at herself about her inability to follow through. Eventually, she leaves the class. Years later, after finishing law school, Marilyn came back to the program and enjoyed almost immediate success.

   When I interviewed Marilyn about the huge gap that existed between her first try and her second, she related that when her husband gave her permission to hire help to raise the children so that she could follow her secretly held desire to continue her education, her personality changed and her depression left her.

   As I queried her, I discovered that prior to going to law school she felt confined and depressed most of the time, and though eager to lose weight, her only real pleasure was food. There are many articles that talk about "eating for the wrong reasons." This is a perfect example.

> When the student
> is ready,
> the teacher
> appears.

Question: ARE YOU EATING FOR THE WRONG REASONS? If you are, resolve that problem first.

2. Sarah — a young woman joined my class because her mother had bought her a gift certificate. She too had problems staying motivated because she really didn't have her own reasons for attending. She enrolled for her mother, a poor reason to begin.

As Sarah and I spoke, she confessed that what she really longed for was a relationship with a young man. Preferably with someone in the law profession because that's where her interests lay. In the same class she met a woman whose son was attending Yale Law School and who was proudly displaying his photograph in the class. When Sarah learned that he was single and the right age for her, she talked to the woman about a possible introduction. After some awkward hesitation, the boy's mother's finally admitted that she didn't think the setup would work because her son only liked slender women.

We had no problem with Sarah after that conversation. The mother of the law student supplied all the incentive Sarah needed. She lost weight and met the young man — a happy ending.

Sarah's mother could not supply the incentive and motivation for Sarah. She needed something else. Motivation: what works for Sarah may not work for Susan.

Question: PROBLEM WITH YOUR MOTIVATION? ASK YOURSELF, WHAT IS THE INCENTIVE THAT WILL WORK FOR YOU?

3. Susie, a young girl, locks herself in a closet because she is terrified of a mouse that's loose in her house. Susie's mother pleads with her to come out, but to no avail. Susie's fear of the mouse is stronger than her desire to leave the closet.

But if a hole is drilled in the closet and a stink bomb is sprayed into the room, does Susie come out of the closet? You just bet she does! Her desire to leave the closet is now stronger than her fear of the mouse.

Question: WHEN BEING MOTIVATED BY SEVERAL THINGS, WHICH MOTIVATOR IS THE STRONGEST? THE STRONGEST ONE WILL WIN.

Motivation follows a happening. Force yourself to do the things that will bring you closer to your goal. Motivation will follow. Avoid your desire to wait for motivation to hit you without any action on your part. But remember and anticipate that you will be more motivated at times than at others. Don't demand perfection of yourself. Keep going, keep doing. Here are some steps for sparking your motivation:

1. Face the Truth

    Admitting a problem involves the necessity of change. The older I get the less I like change. I want what I want without change. In fact, when I think about how much I hate making myself change, I tell myself, "Well, that's just my nature," and that gets me off the hook. If I am 5' 2" I can't be 5' 8", can I?

    But if I'm talking about a habit, it's quite different. I can do something about that. People change spouses by getting divorced. People give up cigarettes, drugs, and alcohol. I can change my eating habits if I choose to. The first step is telling the truth. Facing the truth frees me. Just as in Alcoholics Anonymous, alcoholics must tell the truth about their drinking before they can change, so must overeaters admit their poor eating and exercising habits.

    If you find it difficult to admit your problem with overeating, it may be because you will then have to deal with your discomfort about having a problem in the first place. This, as I have said, is "having a problem about having a problem." Then what would you do about your negative feelings?

Answer: Turn to Chapter 2 and begin to use your Rational Thinking skills.

Force yourself to think of the consequences of remaining as you are, to view yourself as others view you. Think of the ailments you are inviting — the diabetes, the arthritic problems as you age, the increased risk of heart problems, the loss of self-esteem. Then accept slow, moderate change.

Start with small changes. Small changes can very often alter an entire pattern. Suppose you are unaccustomed to eating breakfast. (Most overweights never eat breakfast simply because they ate too much the night before. They wait until they are starving and then watch out!) Begin by making yourself eat breakfast. It can be as little as a small orange, a slice of whole wheat toast, or a 1/4 cup of cottage cheese (see your Getting Started list for other suggestions).

Talk about these changes to others. Each time you talk about it you are reconfirming your intention to continue making changes. You can arrange to tell a friend by phone. If he or she is also having problems, this is an even better arrangement.

2. Read and Reread the Material at the End of this chapter on Self-Talk

Identify and pinpoint what you may be telling yourself that would erode your motivation.

Possible "stinking thinking" could include:

a. *I don't have time to even think about it.*
b. *No matter what I do, it won't work.*
c. *My friend Harriet did all the things you're asking me to do and she is still fat.*
d. *No matter what I do, I'll never find the man or woman of my dreams.*

Responses to these excuses:

a. You could use the time you wail and whine about your weight to begin making changes.

b. You can't prove it won't work. If you eat less and move more, it has to work because weight loss is scientific.

c. I suggest you check out Harriet's records. She may not be telling the truth.

d. You may be right, but you raise the probability of not finding him or her while you are in a size 22.

You will be amazed at the power you have over your behavior. The more forcibly, the more frequently you talk to yourself, the stronger you will become at achieving, at doing, the things you really want to do but find you don't do. Repeat each self-talk statement several times and say it with conviction, with authority. Your response to what you choose to tell yourself will match the authority or lack of authority in your voice as you speak to yourself. Say it passively and your response will be passive — it's that simple. But accepting these statements is not all that simple. If you accept what I am telling you, you will be thinking seriously about doing it. The choice is yours, not mine.

3. Set Realistic Goals

"Wow, I need to give up my goodies, start exercising, keep an eating chart, and what else? I'm overwhelmed already."

It is easy to lose motivation by becoming overwhelmed by the many habits you have to change. "All at once" thinking will fail you in the long run. List your priorities. Refuse to

> Don't prostitute your energies. You Must Prioritize.

work on more than one habit at a time until you've integrated that behavior into your lifestyle. For example, if you have neglected your exercise, you may begin by exercising for a few minutes each day. Once that behavior becomes a habit (the time will vary with each person) and you have learned about your own limits, you will be able to begin incorporating other changes such as counting calories the Living Thin way.

If you can find the discipline to establish small changes in your habits and force yourself to make these changes, the big ones will be easy.

Examples:

- I will make an approximate plan for the day that will include one change of behavior
- I cannot brush my teeth until I have weighed myself in the morning

Create your own penalty and reward system. For example, if you don't snack between meals today, let yourself eat an entire bagel at lunch tomorrow. Or, if you climb two flights of stairs today, permit yourself a cocktail in place of a glass of wine (a difference of 100 calories) tomorrow.

Each one of these suggestions can be used, or changed, in accordance with your personal priorities and preferences. To Live Thin you are going to have to Think Thin.

4. Overcome Procrastination.

Talk about your plan to anyone who will listen. Convert everyone you meet into a support group.

5. Overcome Fatigue and Boredom

These are two of the deadliest destroyers of motivation. When you are tired, avoid eating. Don't even plan for a meal. Either rest or simply keep your mouth closed. For boredom, read the section on boredom in this chapter. I guarantee you won't find it boring.

6. Get Some Exercise

Daily exercise depresses the appetite, relieves boredom and depression, helps you to say "no" more easily, clears the head, and strengthens the backbone. It burns calories too!

Self-Talk

*"Yes, I can find my name on several of these 'stinking thinking' examples, but I find myself, nevertheless, still resisting, still refusing to 'get started.' I enjoy reading, but that's as far as it goes. I know what I need to do, but I still don't feel like doing it. I know you are going to tell me, 'I don't have to FEEL like doing it, I just have to DO IT,' but I **really** don't feel like doing it."*

I promise you that reading alone will not promote change, just as gaining insights into your "stinking thinking" is interesting but still won't give you what you want. Unless you are willing to work and practice, practice and work, nothing will change. No hits, no runs, plenty of errors.

For change of any kind to occur you need to be willing to become a participant. Remaining passive will leave you at square one. My students have taught me that wanting it simply isn't enough. For all these reasons, I am going to give you a simple blueprint for attacking the negative head talk that stops you from taking action. It will motivate you to do the things you need to do.

You, your friends — all of us — are talking to ourselves all the time, continually, automatically. We are barely aware of it. What we choose to tell ourselves about any and all issues causes us to feel as we do. In turn, our feelings motivate our behaviors.

Here is an example. Jane and her roommate Ruth have the same salary and the same job at the same company. One day they are both fired. Jane is depressed and scared. Ruth, on the other hand, has not only accepted it but is looking forward to a better job. Why the disparity? Jane is engaged in negative head talk that goes something like this: *"I wonder what I did or said that was wrong? What if I never find another job?"* With an attitude like that she has an excellent chance of *never* finding another job. Employers are not looking for depressed, scared ladies; neither are potential boyfriends. Ruth, on the other hand, has welcomed the situation and sees it as an opportunity to improve her lifestyle.

Ruth's message to herself and the world is a positive one that will result, in all probability, in a new, more rewarding position. You may ask how Jane can change her negative message to a positive one if she doesn't really feel like it.

The answer is she must be willing to force herself to make statements that are realistic. For example, "Though I don't feel as positive as Ruth does, I know that with my qualifications I will probably find another good job. And I refuse to dwell on the negative aspects of the situation. I am going to immediately make plans to look for other positions."

Each person has the magic, the power within himself, to become his own therapist. By taking action of some kind, or by changing your head talk, you will be putting yourself in charge of whatever situation you may be in.

The fact is that your feelings do not come from what happened but from what you choose to tell yourself about what happened. When you are feeling negative, sad, depressed, angry, guilty or anxious, ask yourself, "What am I saying in my head to cause these feelings?"

Yes, it's true that the thinking is automatic, but challenging your spontaneously occurring head talk is the most effective way

of being able to overcome your "stinking thinking." As you practice, you can deliberately change your thoughts, feelings, and behaviors. When you forcefully "try on" new thoughts, you will
very soon be feeling and behaving in response to your rational
thinking. Here is an example:

Martha is unwilling to even consider making a daily eating
plan. She dislikes being "fenced in." Eating on the run is her
style. Around 4:30 p.m., feeling very hungry, she sees a candy
bar that she really loves. In her head is an automatic message, *"I
am so hungry and that looks so good . . . It's not a big deal, one
candy bar won't make me fat."* She is so right. One candy bar
won't make her fat, but a lack of planning and listening to that
kind of talk is a guarantee for weight gain. Here is a better message: "That candy bar looks delicious, but I will be consuming
400 calories of nothing but garbage (sugar, chocolate) that has
no nutritional value. IT'S NOT WORTH IT! I'll settle for a biscotti, which is approximately 150 calories. It's not a perfect
choice, but it is a much better choice."

What we are talking about here are trade-offs. By changing
her head talk, she arrives at a decision of her own making that
motivates her to make an intelligent choice.

Here's another example: *"Whenever my sister-in-law calls
me she manages to say things that make me feel angry."* Change
that message to, "I refuse to become upset when she insists on
saying things that used to make me angry. She has a right to be
unkind. I can't stop her. I think she enjoys my upsettedness. But
I, in turn, refuse to become upset. We both are making choices.
She is choosing to 'do her thing,' and by refusing to 'should' on
her I will not become upset."

Many people are experts at thinking in negative patterns, and
these negative patterns cause us to behave negatively. That's the
bad news. The good news is that we can actually train ourselves

> **Practice succeeding in your imagination. See yourself where you want to be.**

to think in a positive fashion. The payoffs from overcoming all-or-nothing thinking in all areas of our lives are overwhelming.

I want you to talk to yourself as if you were your own best friend rather than your worst enemy. Here are examples of how the two voices talk to you:

Enemy Within You: *"When I overeat after swearing I would not, it proves that I will always fail and that I simply do not have what it takes."*

Your Own Best Friend: "So I overate. It's not the first time and probably won't be the last time. I've been doing it a long time, but guess what — I refuse to give up on myself. I am determined to take care of the only body I'll ever have. I refuse to live as a victim."

Enemy Within You: *"Getting started today is impossible! I'm just too busy today. I know it will be easier tomorrow, right?"*

Your Own Best Friend: "Wrong! It's always harder tomorrow. Stop looking for excuses and get started. Remember your goal is not perfection, it's simply to get started."

Enemy Within You: *"I have become weary from trying so many different programs. I have so much weight to lose there is no point in getting started. I will never make it."*

Your Own Best Friend: "You can't prove you will never make it. If others can make it, you can make it. Yesterday was yesterday. The worst thing that can happen is that you will fail, and if you do, SO WHAT? You have failed before and survived. Maybe this program is for you. What have you got to lose?"

Self-talk gives you the power to free you from hoping others will be able to provide you with answers. Be absolutely clear about the connection between your thoughts, feelings, and behaviors. Your behavior influences and affects your thinking, and, in turn, your thinking is reflected in your behavior. And the way you feel is affected by both! Thoughts, feelings, and behavior are interconnected. Understanding this, you can begin to use the tools of REBT to be in charge of your own experiences.

This kind of personal self-talk training is exciting, dramatic, and effective. It is another element on the road map that will steer you clear of self-defeating behaviors.

Remember the last time that you really needed to stay away from cookies and you said to yourself, "I am going to really try to give up cookies." Well, I promise that you will not give up cookies. Why? Because your success (and your failures) are determined by the words you choose and the way you say them. In my classes, students are taught that "trying" won't work. Doing is what works. The word itself gives you an excuse. *"Well, I tried. I can't do more than try."* To that I answer, "Oh yes you can. You can do it." Discard the word "try."

> **Discard the word "TRY."**

Another dangerous statement, "I really want to do it" or "I hope I can," needs to be changed to, "It may take time, since I know that changing thinking and behavior habits takes time, but I plan to do more than 'want' to do it. I am going to succeed. I know I can." If you insist on making this statement, your behavior will match it, I promise.

The most common negative head talk you produce is simply, "I just don't feel like doing it." Whatever "it" is, you can immediately superimpose the following message, "I don't have to feel like doing what I have to do, I just have to do it. I'll feel like it later."

Other extremely effective messages include:

1. "I refuse to live like a victim."

2. "Victims are powerless and helpless, and I am determined to take responsibility for taking care of the only body I will ever have."

3. "I am not merely going to 'try' to do better. 'Trying' isn't good enough."

4. "I refuse to feel guilty. If I allow myself to feel guilty, I will overeat."

5. "To lose weight I will not diet. I will find a way that suits me."

6. "I love the concept of trade-offs, both in weight loss and living."

Other self-talk hints:

1. You do not have to have what you think you want if what you want will stop you from reaching your goal.

2. Reading alone will not promote change. You must be willing to work and practice, work and practice.

3. There are slender people who, because of genetics, can go through life without giving up junk food. Don't envy them. Think of the garbage they are pouring into their bodies. Being slender is no guarantee of good health.

4. If you insist on insulting your body with sugar, grease, and foods devoid of nutrients, be prepared to deal with the consequences.

5. Be glad you have the problem and use it as a plus. By giving up white flour, sweets, and grease you will not only lose weight, you will be much healthier. Not a bad exchange.

6. Your goal is not perfection. Your goal is getting started.

7. Your negative head talk is your enemy.

8. How you talk to yourself matters. If you talk to yourself softly and in terms that provide built-in excuses and escape hatches, your response will match your talk. If you talk to yourself with force and authority, you will be in charge of yourself at last.

Self-Acceptance

"I simply don't have what it takes." "I am such an idiot." "I'll never make it." "Others can succeed but I KNOW I can't succeed." This kind of self-talk guarantees failure.

> Don't let yesterday use up today.

"I'll never make it" becomes a self-fulfilling prophesy. No matter what your failures or what you have attempted in the past — these do not mean YOU have failed. You are not what you do. You may be what you eat, but you are not what you do. If your behavior is faulty, it means exactly that. Your behavior, not you, is faulty. And SO WHAT?

If you insist on making statements such as, "I know I can't succeed," I promise that you will not succeed. My students have taught me well. You would rather fail and prove yourself right, than succeed and make a liar out of yourself.

The solution to failure is accepting yourself with all the warts while you use your REBT tools to remind yourself (and others) that it is human to goof up from time to time. Only angels are perfect. Humans are not. It is the "shoulds" in your head that put you into the perfectionists' corner. Chapters 6 and 7 will train you to shed your self-defeating attitudes and behaviors.

Remember, you have a right to avoid losing weight. Refuse to feel guilty. It's your life, and while I am surely not advocating or encouraging your ignoring an overweight problem, I know from experience that you have a right to ignore the problem. You won't be locked up. It's not against the law and, even more important, nothing you do to lose weight will work. At the same time I do want to encourage you to think about the consequences of not losing. If you still are not ready then wait until you are, because change requires commitment. There is no other way.

> **Don't compare yourself to others. Recognize your own strengths.**

What does the word commitment really mean to you? It means you will follow through, no matter what. Example: I am a surgeon. Every Monday I meet with my group to make specific plans and work on changing my eating, thinking, and lifestyle habits. That means I am not available to operate on Monday evenings. Another example, I am pregnant and again my time to work on my health is on Monday evenings. That means I will not deliver my baby on a Monday evening! That is what is meant by a commitment. Be sure you understand what the word means.

Excuses often find their way into self-talk. The reason you even have excuses is because you don't want to make changes. You want to lose weight without making changes. My students taught me everything I know about excuses. One would tell me, *"It's so hard to change or plan because I live alone and living alone makes it difficult to plan a well-balanced meal."* I understand that. The next told me, *"I won't be able to change my habits until I live alone, free of my family's demands."* I understand that too. When I heard one person tell me, *"My mother is in the hospital and that just makes it impossible to make any changes,"* I realized that overweights will make excuses without even realizing the irrational thinking behind them. ANY EXCUSE WILL DO to avoid making changes.

When you hear yourself saying, *"But I don't have the time,"* you're really saying you're not spending the time you do have to do the things you really want to do, such as caring for your health, losing weight, or increasing your self-confidence. Of course you do have the time to take care of the only body you will ever have. Each of us is entitled to 168 hours each week. What separates winners from losers is the way we manage our time. Procrastinators use the classic "not enough time" excuse because they're always thinking it will be easier tomorrow, not realizing that tomorrow it will be harder, not easier.

ASSIGNMENT 2

Now that you know how to attack the junk in your head, let's talk about an assignment for this session. Pick one or more of the following habits (see next page) that have your name on them and tape them on your refrigerator. During the next week or two plan to change one of these habits in keeping with the Living Thin approach. Think gradual. Think moderation. You don't have to be perfect, but DO IT! Combat any negative self-talk with the techniques suggested above. Congratulations! You are on your way to Living Thin.

PINPOINT PROBLEMS AND SITUATIONS
THAT HAVE YOUR NAME ON THEM

1. Eating on the run (No planning)
2. Insufficient exercise

3. Sugars, fats, and salts

4. Portion control

5. Overeating during weekends, travel, or at parties you give or go to

6. Fatigue

7. Boredom, loneliness

8. Eating when upset, angry, frustrated, etc.

Conclusion

Change is extremely difficult. It is so much easier to remain "as is." Change requires a high degree of motivation and energy. When I think about making changes, the thought increases my motivation to resist. I hate change. And yet, change is what I crave, desire, yearn for — oh, the irony! Changing my lifestyle is what I've been dreaming about for a long time. Changing my eating habits, exercise habits, and especially the way I handle stress . . . What to do? What to do?

Read and reread this chapter, which is designed so that you can free yourself from the garbage, the "stinking thinking" that keeps you glued to unhealthy habits. Select the excuses that have your name on them and accept the fact that change begins in your head.

"No one can make you feel inferior without your consent," Eleanor Roosevelt said. Can you see the power of that statement? To accept and incorporate that philosophy leads to inner strength of steel, to total acceptance that each person must own the responsibility of his or her own emotional turmoil whenever it occurs. But even more exciting and important is that if you accept the preceding as true, then you can also see that each person has the ability to fix himself, to alter or eliminate his emotional pain by examining and challenging his foolish head talk.

4

Living Thin Below the Neck

In this chapter:

- The Intelligent Solution to Eating Instead of Dieting
- How Low Calorie Foods Can Make You Fat
- Counting Calories the Living Thin Way
- Designing Your Own Prescription for Permanent Weight Loss
- The Value of a Well-Spent Calorie
- The Art of Intelligent Bingeing
- Living Thin Without Counting Calories
- Becoming an Absolute Snob about Hygiene
- The Value of Exercise

Moving On, Moving Ahead — Ready Yourself for Change

Now that we've taken care of the junk in your head, we can move on. But I need to remind you that we are still talking about changing habits, changing from *thinking habits* to **eating habits**. In this chapter, my goal is to jar you, to motivate you into seeing that without OWNING the material in the chapter, you cannot lose weight for the long haul. The name of the game is learning to eat, not to diet. If you are able to put this chapter into practice, you will have it made.

Along the way we need to ask ourselves repeatedly, "what does it take to change a habit?" Answer: A LOT! Your first job is facing the truth about your habits.

I've learned that many overweights resort to denial as a coping tool. While you have a right to engage in denial if you wish, I promise you if you choose that path, you will live with failure.

Your first task is to recognize your desire to delude yourself about your habits. After you have faced that truth, you need to understand that you have what it takes to make any changes you desire to make. It is simply a matter of your being willing to exercise the emotional muscle required for making those changes.

Begin by making small changes. A marathon runner who starts the race at the head of the pack rarely wins the race. You need to pace yourself by making slow, steady, small changes. The

> The one constant
> of life is change.

problem didn't develop overnight, and it doesn't have to be cured overnight. Being willing to be patient with yourself while you work toward your goal is what is required when changing eating habits. In other words . . . grow up!

How NOT to Choose Calories

When I first became aware of the connection of health and calories to my weight loss, I became obsessive about counting calories. I would eat only low-calorie foods. I began patronizing a company that specialized in low-calorie products. My favorite was a variety of cookie.

Well, it wasn't really a cookie. It was an excuse for a cookie. It was a combination of vanilla flavor and sweetness. The cookie was so light that in order for me to derive full satisfaction, I had to eat the whole bag! The product was promoted as having "ONLY 7 CALORIES PER COOKIE." Each time I ate a cookie, the message in my head was, "It's only seven calories per cookie." I am secretly ashamed that it took me some time to realize that I was consuming about 500 calories per bag. What I also realized was that all this low-cal food was making me fat!

In addition, my good friend, nutritionist Jack Osman, pointed out that very often, low-cal items such as low-cal sour cream or low-cal peanut butter contain chemical substitutes. To save a mere 30 calories I was ingesting chemical additives that might have been detrimental to my health. Not smart.

I also realized that the most important issue related to weight loss was that only overweight people ate low fat, low-cal foods — especially the low-cal foods. You certainly never see a slender person eating low-cal foods. I now practice and preach the virtues of eating like slender people.

This does not preclude, on occasion, eating something low-cal or low fat. I teach and practice a common sense approach that encourages moderation in all habits.

However, making intelligent food choices is predicated on the assumption that you have a rough idea of how many calories you are consuming.

Your goal is to discover approximately how much you can eat to lose, gain, or maintain your weight. It's a numbers game, whether it's money or calories. When you are LIVING THIN, you can have anything you want, provided you can afford it.

What I am about to share with you is all the education you will ever need to take it off and keep it off — healthily, without feeling deprived and having to give up your favorite foods and, above all, without ever feeling hungry.

The key to successful and permanent weight loss is to remind yourself continually to eat frequently. Never let yourself be hungry. If you're hungry, you are not in control of the next bite.

COUNTING CALORIES THE LIVING THIN WAY

"Counting calories is not just the best way to lose weight and keep it off, it's the only way." So said the late, internationally known nutritionist of Tufts University, Dr. Jean Mayer. But it doesn't have to be boring or tedious or even time consuming.

Counting calories is similar to investing in an insurance policy that guarantees your reaching your goal. It enables you to begin eating some foods you never dreamed possible. For example, many calorie conscious people avoid potatoes and spaghetti. But by themselves these foods are fairly low in calories as well as filling and healthy. It's not the potato that makes you fat. We count an average potato as having approximately 100 calories and a large potato, 200. But a pat of butter is 50 calories. So try half of a pat or some ketchup or some other substitute.

Unfortunately, too many people resist any information or knowledge about the scientific issues involved in weight loss. Weight loss is scientific, like the sun rising in the east and setting in the west. When we say it is scientific, we mean that it already has been proven. If I throw myself off the tenth floor of a building, I don't have to agonize about whether I'm going to fall up or down. It's a given.

When you consume approximately 3500 calories less than your body requires to maintain its present weight, you will automatically shed a pound. Conversely, just 50–100 calories per day over your energy needs can put on approximately 10 pounds of fat a year. Let's assume that after a week or two of keeping an eating chart you are maintaining your present weight of 155 lbs. on 1500 calories a day. But let's assume that your cousin Willie comes to live with you, and each evening you enjoy a glass of wine with Willie that heretofore you had not had. Eight ounces of wine is approximately 80 calories. Over a week, you've taken in about 500 calories added to your average weekly caloric intake of 10,500. Over the year you find yourself engaging in this habit for 50 weeks. That means you've added 25,000 calories by having Willie live with you. Doing the math (25,000 divided by 3500) shows that you will gain just over 7 pounds simply from your glass of wine each night.

Conversely, had you been in the habit of drinking a glass of wine the same number of times per year and decided to give up the wine, you would have lost 7 pounds. It's not a question of giving up wine, it's LEARNING what it takes to lose weight, gain weight, and maintain weight, and then engaging in trade-offs.

The reason this approach works is because you are making your own choices, which will vary from time to time. But, regardless of the variations, you will be in charge. THE CHOICES ARE YOURS — that's why it works.

If you're sick and tired of feeling sick and tired about losing and gaining, counting calories is a surefire approach that never misses. For example, in 1994 I went to Russia for about two weeks and lived on a barge. I absolutely could not eat most of the food served to me. Their idea of a delectable American treat was a hot dog roll with a spoonful of applesauce stuck in the middle.

For many days I lived on Snickers bars, knowing full well that each bar contained about 300 calories. But because I knew I could maintain my weight on 1400 calories without starving or gaining weight, I could allow myself, if need be, to eat a candy bar for breakfast, lunch, and dinner and still enjoy the Russian ballet.

Let's return to the fact that weight loss is scientific. Suppose Jane Smith weighs 200 pounds. We have learned that when Jane eats 2000 calories a day, she can maintain her 200 pounds. But when she drops from 2000 to 1000 calories a day, in three and a half days she would have a 3500 calorie deficit and would automatically lose a pound.

Here's how the Living Thin approach to counting calories differs from the others and why, in my opinion, it has been so successful:

1. **It doesn't require you to become a purist** — only eating certain healthy foods, avoiding all others. That's not only boring and tedious, but will guarantee failure.

2. **It doesn't count calories for most vegetables** (other than beans, corn and potatoes). The reason? You are not overweight because you eat too many vegetables. So why bother to count them? The more vegetables you eat the less garbage you will consume.

3. **It keeps calorie counting simple.** Almost any count will do. You could even make up your own number. If you read several books on calories, you will find they all differ. So pick any book that suits you. But avoid making comparisons — it will drive you to the cookie jar. Use round numbers. We don't need to remember that potatoes have 92.5 calories. All moderate sized potatoes are 100 calories, large ones are 200. Sweet potatoes, add 50 calories. It's called the KISS approach — Keep It Simple, Stupid. Use the numbers your book gives for corn and beans.

Dining out counting: Clear soups, 100 calories; Creamed soup, add 100 more. All fish 250 calories, provided it's not fried (sautéed is still 250). Same with chicken.

Counting calories this way and jotting them down helps you develop an awareness of what you are eating, when you are eating, why you are eating, how much you are eating and, let's not forget, THE QUALITY of what you are eating. The higher the quality, the fuller you feel. The fuller you feel, the less you eat. **Lesson to be learned: Never, under any circumstances, allow yourself to feel hungry.**

Warning: If you insist on becoming paranoid about calories, you will fail! I've seen it happen repeatedly. You're better off eating less of something you really enjoy. If your menu consists only of foods you don't enjoy, it won't work. We're not searching for temporary solutions. This is forever.

The Magic of Calories

Why bother to count calories? You have an immediate resistance to doing it. Everyone does. So why bother? There are cases to be made for counting and not counting calories. Let's get to them.

There are literally thousands of books, articles, and programs for controlling your weight. Both you and I have "been there and done that" too many times to count. Still, after so much experience, you still are confused and frustrated. Your confusion actually increases as you age because you have to deal with the various changes of life that occur during your 40s, 50s, 60s and so on.

It all makes for interesting reading and profits for authors, publishers, and salespeople. But "interesting" doesn't translate into effective weight loss, which is THE BOTTOM LINE. At

CALORIES: THE KEY TO WEIGHT LOSS
• Count them as you would your money
• Don't give control of your calories to someone else

some point you simply must ask yourself, "how much can I eat without gaining weight?" THAT QUESTION IS THE START OF GETTING EDUCATED, and the answer is measured in calories.

Think of calories as you would money. Would you want to live in a house or drive a car that you couldn't afford? In our fantasies, most of us would say yes, why not? But are you prepared for the inevitable failure, frustration, guilt and aggravation of such a decision when you lose your house or car? You can see that it is simply a matter of trade-offs. It is the same with food.

Program pushers tell you to only eat when you are hungry. That's ridiculous. Overweight people are hungry all the time. They tell you to eat food that someone else has suggested for you. That's boring, and insulting. You are not a house pet that requires your master to dole out your food to you.

I suggest that you experiment with the only magic bullet you will ever find — yourself and your own educated preferences and decisions. By knowing the approximate caloric value of a small number of food groups, you will be able to make your own decisions. Such a small investment for such a large return.

As for counting calories, as you make these slow but sure changes in your portion control, you will be able to forgo the formal counting and substitute "eyeballing it."

The following simple guide will make understanding calories as simple as learning the names of the continents. There are three basic categories, and all you need to do is keep these ballpark figures in mind. Think of all the time you may have wasted devoting yourself to books, programs, or advice that hasn't worked!

THIS BRIEF LESSON WILL GIVE YOU THE CONTROL AND AMMUNITION NEEDED TO PROCEED, SUCCEED, AND BE IN CHARGE — BECAUSE YOU ARE ASSUMING RESPONSIBILITY FOR YOUR OWN FOOD CHOICES.

200–400 Calories

Poultry — Count 4 ounces of poultry prepared without the skin or any fat added as 200 calories.

Meat — Nearly all 4 ounce servings fit into this range. Lean cuts are about 250 and fatty ones like short ribs are 400.

Fish — Count 200 calories for 4 ounces of unfried fish, without added butter.

Pies/Cakes — Figure 300 calories for fruit pies, 200 for plain cake and 400 for frosted cake.

100–200 Calories

Cheese, Milk and Ice Cream — Count 100 calories for 1 ounce of most hard cheeses. One cup of whole milk is 160 calories; skim milk is 90. Half a cup of ice cream is 150 calories.

Cereals & Grains — Count all unsweetened cereals as 100 calories per 1 ounce serving. Pasta is 190 calories for each 1 cup serving, cooked, without sauce. Add 30 calories for plain tomato sauce and 150 for meat sauce.

0–100 Calories

Eggs — Count 80 calories for a plain egg.

Cream & Yogurt — Count 50 calories for 1 tablespoon of most types of cream including sweet, whipped and sour. Low fat plain yogurt is 10 calories per tablespoon.

Potatoes — Average size counts as 100 calories. Large counts as 200 calories. Sweet potato adds 50 calories.

Fruits — Apples, pears, and bananas are 100 calories each. Grapefruits and oranges are 50 calories each. Peaches, wedges of melon or pineapple, and a half cup of berries are 30 calories each.

Breads — Count 80 calories per slice of whole wheat or seven grain bread. Avoid white flour except for bagels if you love them. Large bagels are 350–400 calories each. Small (frozen type) count for 180 calories each. Rolls and muffins are 150 calories each. Crackers are 25 calories.

Beverages — Coffee and tea are zero. The average mixed drink is 150–200 calories. About sodas — even diet sodas, which contain a lot of sodium and cause water weight retention — the less said and the less indulged in the better. 80 calories for a glass of wine (at a party or just to save calories, mix half-and-half with Perrier: 40 calories). Beer is 125 calories per 8 ounces. Nonalcoholic beers are often one-third the calories of the alcoholic brews.

Fats & Oils — Count all butter, margarine, shortening and oils at 100 calories per level tablespoon. Same for mayonnaise, Russian dressing, and tartar sauce.

DON'T REMOVE TOO MANY CALORIES FROM YOUR DIET. AVOID FEELING DEPRIVED.

Vegetables — Count as zero. Exceptions: potatoes, beans and corn.

Whispers & Dashes (of mayo or sour cream) — NO CHARGE!

What It Takes Regardless of Height, Age, or Genetics, to Lose Weight

People have preconceived ideas on what it takes to lose weight, and they very often use them as excuses. Do genetics make a difference? Of course. It's part of everyone's formula. Some people have a naturally slow metabolism.

Genetics do make a difference. One baby can't stop being in motion, the other is rarely in motion. You may be in between these two extremes. And — here is how unpredictable genetics are — you may have the inclination to not move AND STILL HAVE A SNAPPY METABOLISM.

If, however, you are the kind of person who is not inclined to move AND have a sluggish metabolism (a double whammy), that does not mean you can't be thin. It means you have to want it enough to do more to get what you want and force yourself to overcome your genetic bent.

The double whammy can still have a silver lining, though. You can choose to see this as a plus rather than as a minus. By making healthy food choices and moving more, you will increase the probability of having more energy, aging more slowly, and living a longer and better life.

My friend Irwin has a jazzy metabolism. He can eat all the junk he desires and his trousers are still loose. He also has a heart problem. Do I envy him? Absolutely not! You and I are going to have to eat healthily if we want to take it off and keep it off. Irwin has no desire to lose weight. He justifies his taste for garbage as an excuse to gain weight.

Even if you have a slow metabolism, you can still make it a plus for yourself. The choice is yours.

One of my dear friends is a stoic individual if ever there was one. If nature had her way, she would have been an attractive and probably overweight woman. Her very sluggish metabolism made it very easy for her to gain weight very quickly. But this woman embodies the essence of what I am teaching in this program: that you can have what you want if you are willing to pay your dues. After experimenting with a number of approaches for weight loss that simply didn't work, she finally accepted the fact that the only way she would get what she wanted was to increase her exercise.

She found an exercise tape that appealed to her and committed herself to exercising for thirty minutes before work every day. That meant she had to get up at 6:00 instead of 6:30. Can you guess the results? She not only achieved the weight she wanted but she also raised her muscle tone, energy level, and appearance of radiance.

You see how my friend converted a minus into a plus? She did it by concentrating on exercise and nutrition. This is a formula for good health we should be teaching from cradle to grave. Whether you are 10 years old or 90 years old, concentrating on exercise and nutrition is what good health is all about.

Designing Your Personal Prescription For Permanent Weight Loss

My second class of Living Thin included the following examples of how easy it is to subtract calories without having to feel deprived or hungry.

Counting Calories Your Way

Breakfast 7:30 a.m.		*Calories*
8 oz. orange juice		110
2 fried eggs with 2 pats of butter		230
1 croissant with 1 pat of butter		270
coffee with cream & sugar		30
	Total	640

Morning Snack 10 a.m.		
doughnut (yeast-glazed)		235
coffee with cream & sugar		30
	Total	265
	Grand Total	905

Counting Calories The Living Thin Way

Breakfast 7:30 a.m.		*Calories*
1 orange (more filling)		60
2 eggs (soft boiled or poached)		160
2 slices 7-grain bread		160
1 tsp. Sorrell jam		14
coffee (black)		0
	Total	394

Morning Snack 10 a.m.		
veggies (carrots, etc.)		Free
tea or coffee (black)		0
	Total	0
	Grand Total	394

Comparison
    Breakfast & Snack Your Way   905
    Breakfast & Snack Living Thin Way   394
                      Savings 511

Counting Calories Your Way

Lunch 12:45 p.m.   *Calories*

	Calories
tuna salad on rye bread	690
6 oz. oil-packed tuna	(330)
2 Tbsp. mayo*	(200)
2 slices rye bread	(160)
10 potato chips	105
1/7 of 9" apple pie	345
coffee with cream & sugar	30
Total	1170

Afternoon Snack

small candy bar	300
Total	300
Grand Total	1470

* Mayo: 100 calories for 1 level Tbsp.; when salad is prepared in restaurant, allow twice as much mayo calories.

Counting Calories The Living Thin Way

Lunch 12:45 p.m.		*Calories*
turkey sandwich		228
3 slices breast meat		
2 slices 7-grain bread		
lettuce, tomato & mustard		
banana		100
coffee (black)		0
	Total	328

Afternoon Snack		
small apple		60
handful of plain sunflower seeds		25
	Total	85
	Grand Total	413

Comparison

Lunch & Snack Your Way		1470
Lunch & Snack Living Thin Way		413
	Savings	1057

Counting Calories Your Way

Dinner 6 p.m.		*Calories*
1 cup minestrone soup		100
sirloin steak (5 oz.)		550
10 French fries cooked in vegetable oil		160
salad w/ 2 Tbsp. Russian dressing		200
slice of plain pound cake		300
coffee with cream & sugar		30
	Total	1340

Late Night Snack		
ice cream bar		350
	Total	350
	Grand Total	1690

Counting Calories The Living Thin Way

Dinner 6 p.m.		*Calories*
1 cup vegetable soup		70
veal cutlet (5 oz.)		300
baked potato w/ 1 pat butter		135
salad w/1 tsp. low-cal dressing		12
asparagus		Free
small roll w/ 1 pat butter		135
slice of plain pound cake		300
coffee (black)		0
	Total	952

Late Night Snack		
Alba shake made w/ skim milk		117
	Total	117
	Grand Total	1069

Comparison
Dinner & Snack Your Way	1690
Dinner & Snack Living Thin Way	1069
Savings	621

Comparison: YOUR WAY v. LIVING THIN

		Calories
Breakfast & Snack Your Way		905
Breakfast & Snack Living Thin Way		394
	Savings	511
Lunch & Snack Your Way		1470
Lunch & Snack Living Thin Way		413
	Savings	1057
Dinner & Snack Your Way		1690
Dinner & Snack Living Thin Way		1069
	Savings	621
Total One Day Savings		2189

In one week, Your Way gains you 5 extra pounds. Your choice — Healthy choices and counting calories — or mindless eating?

How to Triple Your Dinner Calories[1]

Calories		Added Fats/Sugar	Total Fat Adjusted Calories
20	lettuce & tomato salad	+ 1 Tbsp. mayo (100) =	120
60	whole wheat bread	+ 1 pat butter (35) =	95
35	broccoli (1/2 cup)	+ 1½ oz. Hollandaise sauce (180) =	215
150	3 oz. chicken breast (deskinned)	+ gravy (100) =	250
100	baked potato (med.)	+ 1 pat butter + s-cream (35 + 100) =	235
90	8 oz. skim milk	+ whole milk (60) =	150
100	baked apple (for dessert)	+ Replace with apple pie =	410

Total Calories 1475

The response of students to these examples was always the same. They were stunned by the simplicity of the message in the charts. They saw that by simply making a number of tiny changes in their meal plans, a huge difference was made in their calorie intake and their chances of succeeding in taking off weight.

When we talk about finding your personal prescription, it will include: 1) How much and what you can eat to lose, gain, or maintain your weight; and 2) How much exercise you will do.

You will test your data by weighing yourself daily, with the understanding that as you age you need to eat less and move more. It also involves discovering foods you find to be nutritious and delicious.

By keeping an eating chart and experimenting with some daily exercise, you will learn in approximately one or two weeks how much you can eat and how much you need to move in order to lose, gain, or maintain weight. Once you know this number you are on your way to being in charge. Don't be afraid to experiment. Above all — AVOID RIGIDITY. It will become tedious and boring and IT WON'T WORK.

If you walk into any bookstore or look at your own books, you will find handsomely bound books with beautiful covers related to weight loss, with more being published almost daily. Reading closely you find that each one relies on the same basic plan for everyone — short or tall, young or old, rich or poor, a formula that promises to be all things to all people. Such programs wind up being nothing to anybody in particular.

Your own, one-of-a-kind, unique formula for losing, gaining, or maintaining weight will probably be different from everyone else's. SO AVOID MAKING COMPARISONS. As Shakespeare said in *As You Like It,* they are odious. Would a middle-aged woman suffering from depression eat the same way as a twenty-year-old woman who just delivered her first born child? Would an active teenager eat the same way as a bank manager? Would a construction worker eat the same way as a librarian?

Living Thin advocates that each person design an eating and living plan that works for that individual. Not one that works for his or her cousin, co-worker, or spouse. John and Mary, for

---

No set of rules works for everyone;
Knowing what you want is 50% of the battle.

example, live together and are very compatible sexually and temperamentally, but they have entirely different eating tastes. Allowances for these differences have to come into their eating plans.

YOUR GOAL IS TO FIND A PLAN THAT WILL WORK FOR YOU. You are on your way to feeling better physically, mentally and emotionally. You will love the journey, I promise.

Sylvia's Personal Prescription:
How She Loses, Maintains, or Gains

Maintenance — approximately 1400 calories.

For Weight Loss (approx. 1–1.5 pounds per week) — 1200 calories

Let's PLAN a day that will allow Sylvia to go to dinner for one of her favorite meals.

BREAKFAST

1/2 grapefruit	50 calories
1 cup oatmeal with skim milk	100 calories
1 slice of toast with 1/2 pat butter	100 calories
BREAKFAST TOTAL	250 Calories

LUNCH

3 oz. turkey on whole wheat bread with lettuce
and tomato (with whisper of mayo)

OR

Huge salad (romaine lettuce, carrots,	
sliced turkey, and light dressing)	220 calories
Apple	100 calories
Cup of tea or coffee	0 calories
LUNCH TOTAL	320 Calories

SNACK

1 rice cake	50 calories

4 – 6 glasses of water throughout the day

DINNER

Manhattan cocktail	165 calories

(worth every calorie because I love manhattan cocktails. I learned that the pleasure of drinking manhattans increased a thousandfold as I followed the Living Thin philosophy.)

Cup of vegetable soup	100 calories
3 oz. broiled or sautéed fish	200 calories
Baked potato with 1 tsp.	
sour cream	150 calories
Assorted vegetables	FREE
DINNER TOTAL	615 calories

DAY'S TOTAL	**1215 CALORIES**

My Living Thin philosophy has taught me how to "have it all." You can too!

Small Changes in Your Thinking and Daily Food Choices Result in Considerable Weight Loss (or Gain)

Mary has three cups of coffee a day. Three cups of coffee with approximately 1/3 cup of whole milk equals 75 calories. One-third of a cup of skim milk equals 25 calories. The difference in one day is 50 calories. Let's check it out: Fifty calories seven days a week equals 350 calories. Fifty-two weeks in a year equals 18,200 calories.

In two years Mary has added 36,400 additional calories by using whole milk instead of skim milk. By substituting skim milk for whole milk, she will lose or gain 5 pounds of fat each year or 10 pounds in two years.

Freeing You From Your "Diet Mentality"

Irene has lost her weight and is now on maintenance. Her only concern is keeping off the weight she took off. One night a week Irene enjoys going to Denny's after a night at the theater and sharing dessert. A slice of hot apple pie with a scoop of REAL vanilla ice cream (approximately 300 calories per person).

By eating it slowly, she will derive as much pleasure as she would have during her former "fat" days.

Irene is learning she can "have it all" but not "all the time," the same thinking that separates mature people from immature people.

Getting More Pleasure for Your Calories

Before Irene's Living Thin days, she and Susie, who was very slender, both would order a deli sandwich. Irene would finish her sandwich in half the time as Susie. Irene also had only half the pleasure. Let's analyze why Irene was getting the worst of both worlds.

Very often a major difference between slender people and fat people is the rate at which they consume their food. Overweight people barely finish one bite before they are loading up for the next one. Conversely, slender people tend to chew their food, savor their food before they swallow it.

When you eat slowly the feeling of satisfaction increases immeasurably. In other words, a rapid eater has to eat twice as much to feel as satisfied as a slow eater would.

By increasing your awareness of fast eating vs. slow eating, you will have the BEST of both worlds — you will enjoy your food more and eat less.

Calories are like people — we are all equal, but some of us are more equal than others. George Orwell used a similar premise for his well-known novel *Animal Farm*, in which all the animals were supposedly equal, but the animals (and the reader) very soon discovered that the animals with the power to make decisions were "more equal" than the rest. The same can be said about calories. Even though all calories are equal in their energy producing ability, whether they are protein, carbohydrate, or fat, the effects these substances have on the body vary greatly. For this reason, fat, carb, or protein foods have different value when you are trying to lose weight.

Here is a simple description to help in your understanding of what is different about protein foods, carbohydrate foods, and fat foods and how each relates to counting calories, weight loss, your overall health, and the aging process.

Protein Foods

(1 gram of protein = 4 calories)

Protein is required in the diet because it is the structural core of the body. It might be called the "stuff of life." Protein is essential for the growth, repair, and the formation of new tissue. It is also a source of energy.

Sources of protein include dairy products, fish, fowl, beef and pork, and the plant sources, which are now almost universally accepted as equal or superior to the animal sources: legumes, grains, soy products, and fruit and vegetables in a variety.

For the purpose of counting calories to lose weight, it is important to remember that each gram of protein is worth 4 calories. If you are on a crash diet, your body will deplete stored protein that is needed by the body to repair itself. This is a reason to avoid crash diets.

In other words, 1 gram of protein equals 4 calories. Your body uses it for repair and maintenance.

Carbohydrates — Simple and Complex

(1 gram of carbohydrates = 4 calories)

Carbohydrates fall into two groups: Simple Carbohydrates — pies, cookies, ice cream, candy, and all refined sugar.

Complex Carbohydrates — potatoes, corn, all grains such as rice, wheat and barley, fruit, beans, and breads. Fruit, while sweet, is nutritionally desirable because it contains fiber and in many cases is packed with vitamins and minerals.

Some weight loss programs actually abolish carbohydrates. I believe that is unrealistic because of the difficulty and undesirability of sustaining such a diet. Taking off weight has to be done in a manner that is not only healthy but also "livable."

However, I do suggest cutting down, not cutting out carbohydrates while you are losing weight. I have found from working on myself and others that when we limit (not eliminate) fruit, grains, breads, and legumes, it is easier to lose and maintain our weights.

My theory, based on personal experience and my observations of others, is that by practicing a moderate, but balanced, set of choices daily, we are getting the results we want. You can increase the carbohydrates once you have reached maintenance.

So, 1 gram of carbohydrates equals 4 calories. Your body uses it for immediate energy. Cut back, but not out, on carbohydrates when trying to lose weight.

Fat Foods

(1 gram of fat = 9 calories) — more than twice as much as protein and carbohydrates

Example: One lamb chop equals 220 calories, 135 of which come from fat, whereas two skinless chicken breast halves equal 280 calories, of which only 54 come from fat.

THINK about the differences! Two chicken breast halves, deliciously prepared or a single lamb chop. Think in terms of health, eating pleasure, feeling full and satisfied. For the intelligent solution — you tell me.

Another example: 1 almond without oil or salt equals 7 calories. However, 1 Brazil nut equals 28 calories. Are all nuts equal? Definitely not.

Does knowing so make it easier to decide which is a good snack? Definitely. You can have a very satisfying snack of 10 almonds and 1 apple and consume only 130 calories. The math is simple. The difference between the choices is nearly 300 calories.

So, calories are not about being hungry or giving up your favorite foods. Calories are simply about educating your head so you know where your bread is buttered, so to speak.

Small fat changes make big differences. By leaving out 1 teaspoon of fat every day for six months, you can save yourself about 2.25 pounds of fat.

Wait. Before you decide to give up your fat life, remember your Living Thin philosophy of exercising common sense and moderation. Some fat is crucial for your good health. No matter who you are, you need approximately 80 calories of fat each day. We don't want those joints to dry out.

Most of the fat you eat is hidden in food as part of what you normally eat (mayonnaise, for example). It may be added to a low fat food to flavor it up (butter on a potato or dressing on a salad, which makes 90 percent of the calories in the salad).

How can you GAIN weight easily? Eat at a salad bar! One tablespoon of salad dressing equals approximately 100 calories. A few scoops from the ladle could pack a huge calorie punch. These little ladles look innocent but each carries about 2 ounces, which could cost you 100 CALORIES PER OUNCE. Two ladles and you have 400 CALORIES. However, you could have your dressing on the side and dip each forkful into the dressing for the same flavor and SAVE CALORIES BY THE HUNDREDS!

How to Eat More and Weigh Less
1 lamb chop = 220 calories
15 grams FAT
135 calories from FAT!

2 half chicken breasts = 280 calories
6 grams FAT
54 calories from FAT!

It is a wonderful way to get the flavor at home or when eating out. Or you may switch to a low fat dressing. Another intelligent option is to add some water to the thick dressing and pour it over your salad. You get the flavor running all over the salad rather than concentrated on just a few bites.

There are other calorie and fat bombs at the salad bar. Be sure to LIMIT, NOT ELIMINATE, your portions of grated cheese, olives, bacon bits, and avocado. Avoid winding up with a salad that is low-cal and tasteless — IT WON'T WORK.

Let's say I have a 300 calorie Snickers bar in one hand and 300 calories of oil in a cup in the other hand. If I had a choice of spending 300 calories on the candy bar or using the oil if I am trying to lose weight, which would I choose?

Answer — the Snickers bar. Because the oil provides no feeling of fullness and the candy bar will, at least for a period of time, hours perhaps. The oil simply is "dressing" and though it does provide flavor, it adds nothing in terms of bulk. While I don't advocate eating candy all the time, and I have no intention of drinking the oil, the point is about seeing the better of two evils when faced with difficult and limited choices.

On a maintenance diet, when I choose a candy bar or a portion of ice cream and pie, it is twice as satisfying because in my mind I know that I am still controlling my calories.

If you usually consider the salad bar your only option when it comes to lunch, you may want try a sandwich for a change. Despite what you may think, a sandwich is a wonderful choice. You can make it from two slices of whole grain bread, thick slices of tomato, romaine lettuce, onion, sprouts, and a spread of mayo or honey mustard dressing and the calorie count is only around 350.

Again, 1 gram of fat equals 9 calories, more than twice as much as protein and carbohydrates contain. But don't be foolish;

some fat is required for good health. Watch out for those hidden fats!

Nibbling and Noshing: Your Way vs. the Living Thin Way

Your Way — Mindless Eating Between Meals

> Time: 10:30 a.m. Half (jelly-wheat) Doughnut and Coffee
> Place: Office
> Thoughts: "I see it; I want it . . . Big Deal! Besides, it's healthy."
> Calories: 80

> Time: 2:30 p.m. 1.8 oz. Baby Ruth candy bar
> Place: Office
> Thoughts: "My lunch was drab . . . didn't enjoy it. I refuse to sit here and watch others eating that delicious candy bar that was passed around this afternoon."
> Calories: 260

> Time: 5:30 p.m. martini and 4 oz. shelled hickory nuts
> Place: Home
> Thoughts: Waiting for dinner
> Calories: 763

> Time: 9–11 p.m. 6 saltines and 5 1-oz. cubes of assorted cheeses
> Place: Home
> Thoughts: Watching TV
> Calories: 590

> Total for the day: 1693 calories

Nibbling and Noshing the Living Thin Way

Time: 10:30 a.m. Coffee or tea or hot water and
lemon instead of the half doughnut for 80 calo-
ries
Place: Office
Thoughts: "I'm not hungry; why waste calories?"
Calories: 0

Time: 2:30 p.m. 6 almonds and a small apple in-
stead of the candy bar that costs 260 calories
Place: Office
Thoughts: "I enjoy a snack at this time"
Calories: 116

Time: 5:30 p.m. Perrier with ice and lime with
dip and veggies or marinated veggies instead
of a cocktail and nuts that cost 763 calories
Place: Home
Thoughts: Waiting for dinner
Calories: 30

Time: 9–11 p.m. Before retiring I can have a 100
calorie snack — Chocolate Alba with milk instead of the cheese and crackers that cost 590
calories
Place: Home
Thoughts: "I had a full course dinner. I can wait
for my snack."
Calories: 117

Total calories for the day: 263 instead of 1693

Difference for One Day of Nibbling and Noshing:

1693
–263
1430 calories

1430 x 5 (workdays) = 7150 calories or 2 lbs. in
5 days from snacks — 5 DAYS ONLY!

THE ART OF INTELLIGENT BINGEING:
Learning to Cope with Binges

Plan A Binge

Let's say you have a party to go to on Saturday evening at which you expect to see alcoholic beverages, rich appetizers, entrees, and desserts. You just know what is going to happen when you find yourself conversing and nibbling and losing track of your calorie count. Here is what I suggest:

Three days before the party, start by cutting your daily caloric intake by 100 calories. Let's say you are on a 1200 calorie schedule. You will cut back to 1100 to save some calories for the party. How do I do it? I can do it by omitting a slice of bread with butter or by eating just a sandwich and a half instead of two. One less banana will knock off 100 calories. A little less dressing on a salad will save approximately 100 calories. That's all you need to do for the three days leading up to the party.

During the days leading up to the party, I recommend you plan your binge. Make yourself a menu. It will look like this:

Two glasses of wine — 160 calories

Hors d'oeuvres — I choose to have 300 calories
   worth.

One portion each of roast beef (one slice) and
shrimp — 400 calories, combined.
As many vegetables as I want; they are free.
A roll with butter — 150 calories.
A generous portion of fruit mold — 100 calories.
A final glass of wine — 80 calories.

Total — just under 1200 calories.

The natural inclination is to say to yourself that you've ru-
ined your meal plan by having eaten too much at the party. This
tendency to feel guilty about eating at the party is what ruins the
best laid plans. You just cannot stand the guilt feelings, so you
decide to give up. So you go back to square one — overweight
and not doing anything about it, figuring you'll find some kind
of diet later.

But I learned better. I educated myself to think differently. I
back up and say, "Wait a minute. For breakfast and lunch combined I took in 500 calories. I had 1200 at the party and now I'm
at 1700 for the day. Actually, I'm only 500 calories over my budget. That isn't so much. It certainly isn't as bad as it feels. I had a
good time at the party, and, oh yes, I forgot about the 300 calories I saved. So REALLY, I'm only over by two hundred calories. When I think about that and the fun I had at the party, I
don't mind cutting back on Sunday and Monday by 100 calories
each. In fact, that'll be easy.

This is the pattern of behavior of slender people. They do it
without even knowing it. When you begin behaving like one of
them, you will become more like them. Overweight people do the
reverse. Luckily you are not behaving like a fat person any more.

Now about THE UNPLANNED BINGE. Let's say I'm on
1000 calories a day, and I've already eaten my 1000. My husband informs me that his business partner has arrived in town at

8 p.m., and we are going out with him. Thank God they have already eaten.

I have two bourbons that cost me about 220 calories each and a snack of nuts that costs me anywhere from 20–50 calories. We go to the deli and I have a corned beef sandwich that costs me 350 calories and a coke for 100 calories. That is a total of 940 calories.

Here is how the day looks now. My 1000 calories plus the extra 940. That puts me up to just under 2000 calories — 1000 over budget.

The first thing to do is to avoid panicking. And a crucial issue is to not, repeat, NOT, skip breakfast. Skipping that next meal is the natural and easy thing to do after a binge. However, if you do skip, you are setting yourself up for another binge later in the day. Instead, cut back by about 100 calories daily for a week to make up for the excess. Additionally, you can increase your exercise moderately by 2–4 minutes each day for a week.

After the binge, the first three days of cutbacks are easy because the memory of the binge is fresh in mind. The next three to four days are tougher. But through it all, I have an image in my head that sustains me — that I am really learning to have it all. What does that mean here?

It means if I'm willing to pay back, I can have a binge. I don't have to panic at the thought. And as I pay back, I am improving my discipline skill gradually without too much effort.

Knowing that I can occasionally have a binge is one of the major reasons for the success of this program. I'm thinking with much joy about having had a delicious bread pudding at Cafe Bijou here in Sarasota, Florida, a few days ago. Worth every calorie, plus! You too can occasionally enjoy bread pudding at Cafe Bijou after you have learned to Live Thin.

SYLVIA'S MIDDLE-OF-THE-NIGHT BINGE

While teaching Living Thin, I had a middle-of-the-night eating experience that became an important part of my program. I'd wake up feeling hungry with an overwhelming urge to eat a lot — to stuff myself with something enjoyable to my heart's content. As I look back on it now, I know that my body was rebelling against the changes I was making in my eating habits. This is another reason for making GRADUAL CHANGES.

Now back to my overwhelming hunger. Being a "sweet-aholic," I naturally thought of something sweet. Perhaps cake with ice cream. By now I had learned that sweets are out. If I had the sweets, I'd have to give up on the program. However, that does not eliminate everything I enjoy. When you make this type of statement to yourself, be sure to say it with authority and conviction. You will find that strong talk works.

I can't have sweets, but how about a toasted bagel with a slice of cheese with a whisper of mayo? Remember, there is no charge for whispers. And then some coffee. That's it. Then I have the bagel and coffee, and then I say, "Is that enough?" My answer is, "NO. I WANT MORE. I WANT TO FEEL STUFFED." Then I say to myself, "If you want it that much, have it." The result? Three toasted bagels with cheese and coffee. "Do you feel satisfied now?" Finally, the answer is "YES." This is a gift you have given yourself. Be sure to enjoy it.

Now be brave and count the damage. The three bagels at 160 calories each comes to 480 calories for the bagels (important to note that these were Lenders bagels, not the very large 300–400 calorie jobs). Six slices of real cheese is 100 calories each, making 600. The whisper of mayo carries no charge, because whispers are free. So the total is 1080 calories.

1. Count up the calories and find out how far over you went. In this case, let's assume your daily allotment is 1200 calories and your night binge was 1100. You have gone over by 1100 calories.

2. Your natural inclination is to skip breakfast, especially after a binge that is 1100 calories over your scheduled intake. You say to yourself, "I need to make up 1100 calories to avoid gaining weight." Instead, plan to drop to 1000 calories for the first three days. This is rather easy because the memory of the binge is still fresh in your mind, and some of it is still in your stomach. Remember, you are not to skip a meal and "go on a diet." That is not part of this plan. Simply, plan your meal in accordance with a 1000 calorie a day plan. And remember, we are not counting most vegetables. And plan to increase your exercise by 2–3 minutes a day.

3. You have taken care of 600 calories. Good for you. For the next three to four days drop 100 calories to the 1100 calorie level. Continue with the slight increase in exercise. Now you have accomplished something quite amazing.

You had your 1000 calorie binge when you really needed it. You did not starve or diet for the next week. You simply cut down on calories slightly and increased exercise slightly. At the end of the week, you will probably not only have eliminated the extra calories, but may even have lost weight. And best of all, you will have seen that you can have a big binge without gaining weight, and you are developing discipline habits that will serve you well forever and a day.

By making an intelligent effort in the present, the future automatically improves. Reversing old eating habits takes time. When you reverse them and own your new habits, you will love it.

Measuring Success

If you are accustomed to bingeing several times a week and you are now only bingeing only twice a week, that is success. Each person has to accept his own style, his own tempo. Some people will change more quickly than others. Avoid counting or comparing. No one-upmanship please. Accept yourself AS IS. Avoid people who want you to be what you are not — unless it's your stockbroker and he is doing a fantastic job.

Gradual change is your goal. You do not have to be a size 8 for your daughter's wedding! You will be practicing these skills for life so why hurry. Being in charge is so much fun. The choice is yours.

"If I could recommend just one thing to someone who wants to lose weight and be in control, it would be to keep a food diary." So says John F. Foreyt, Ph. D. and director of the Nutrition Research Clinic at Baylor College of Medicine in Houston. "People who are willing to keep food diaries will succeed. Those who are unwilling will fail."

ASSIGNMENT 3

1. The best way to learn to deal with a binge is to deal with a binge. So go ahead and PAB — Plan A Binge.
2. Examine the pluses and minuses of keeping an eating chart. The minus is, it's a PITA (Pain In The Ass). The pluses are as follows:
   A. It will never lie to you unless you lie to it.

B. It will educate you.

C. Whenever you are in doubt you can turn to your eating chart.

D. It is the best ally you will ever have.

Remember to avoid changing your mind about keeping an eating chart. Rather, concentrate on changing your attitude about keeping an eating chart.

THE GOOD AND BAD NEWS
ABOUT COMPULSIVE EATING

"When I start, I can't stop."

The bad news is you've been compulsive a long time, and it won't go away immediately. The good news is you can beat it. Sylvia was and still is compulsive about eating.

Also good news is that you don't have to stop. You merely have to learn to control and harness. By accepting your compulsive nature you are free to modify it. You are not required to stop. What is needed is the awareness and acceptance that you are what you are. That is the freedom to be who and what you are.

More good news — being compulsive doesn't mean you are an emotional wreck. It could mean that at times you are, but it definitely means that, like Sylvia, you are compulsive by nature. Creative people are often compulsive. Being compulsive has many positive attributes. Keep them!

Success in life comes not from holding a good hand, but in playing a poor hand well.

Warren G. Lester

I disagree with so many self-help books that tell you that to be okay you have to get rid of who you are. Your essence is holy; you should never listen to anyone who says different.

Don't give up. Compulsive people are not "giver-uppers." That's a big plus! A major problem, however, is immoderation. By disciplining yourself to exercise moderation, you can harness your compulsivity and make it work for you.

Understand, there are psychological and chemical factors that may exacerbate your compulsivity — chocolate and sugar products, for instance, which cause your pancreas to spill insulin and results in your appetite being stimulated and you being hungry. Just smelling sweets triggers an irresistible desire to indulge. I suggest you read carefully the information on sugar, which is coming up in the next chapter.

Slender people can eat sugar and nothing happens, whereas an overweight, compulsive personality doesn't have the luxury. Most people who are overweight turn to sweet foods when they are upset. Those of you who respond in this way should return to Chapter 2 and brush up on your Rational Thinking skills. Unless you are the captain of your ship and can control your emotional responses, you are destined to turn to overeating just as an alcoholic turns to alcohol, a gambler to gambling, a druggie to drugs, or shoppers to the mall.

The Solutions

1. First tell the truth. Accept that you have a compulsive personality. And accept that CHANGE NEEDS TO BE GRADUAL.

2. Watch your Low Frustration Tolerance. You are not going to control your compulsive nature in six minutes. Refuse to be compulsive about being compulsive.

3. Watch your perfectionism. Feel free to goof, experiment, and learn. The need to be perfect prevents you from learning new behaviors.

4. Have a plan.

In summary, learn to accept your compulsive nature as Sylvia does hers. The control comes from having a plan. When I am at goal weight, I allow myself to eat compulsively on occasion. And do I enjoy it! YES, I ABSOLUTELY REFUSE TO FEEL GUILTY. I am willing to assume responsibility. When I eat compulsively, I do it deliberately. I tell myself that I have earned the right to eat compulsively — on occasion. That is what we mean when we say that "discipline sets you free."

It's okay to be compulsive. You just can't be compulsive all the time. Grow up and fight your LFT every inch of the way. (That is the real fight!)

Avoid perfectionism. Having unrealistic expectations for yourself and others places you in a constant state of stress. There is negative and positive stress. DISTRESS, the negative type, pushes your compulsive buttons.

Switching your focus from the size of your body to the health of your body will motivate you to deal with the real issues of health.

5

Your Health, Living Young, and Exercise

AGING

Many years ago, my views on aging were greatly influenced by two books written by Gaylord Hauser, *Mirror, Mirror On The Wall* and *Gaylord Hauser's Treasury of Secrets*. Hauser was a famous nutritionist in his day, much of whose work was done in Europe with movie stars from Hollywood and other world-famous personalities who could afford the luxury of focusing their attention on longevity and "the good life."

I remember thinking how motivated those actors and actresses must have been. After all, their careers depended on their health and appearance. I have taught every student of Living Thin to be as big a snob about their body as was Gloria Swanson in her day.

Over the years (including two major fires and moving half a dozen times) I've lost art, clothing, and jewelry but have never

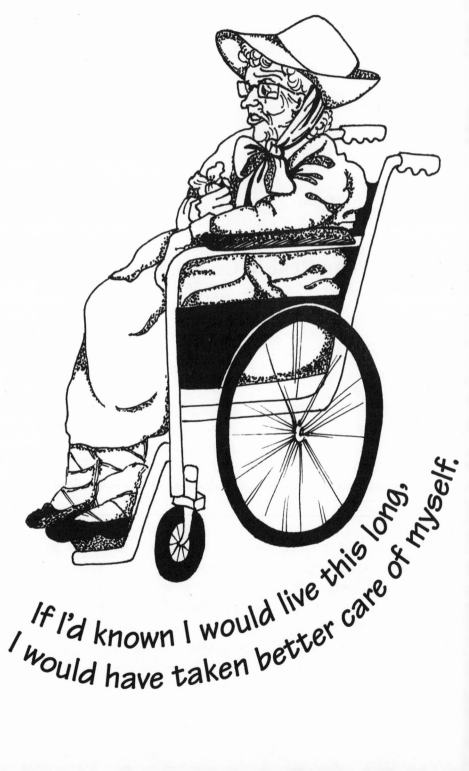

If I'd known I would live this long, I would have taken better care of myself.

let go of Hauser's books, which are, unfortunately, no longer in print. These books concern themselves with the benefits of maintaining your outward appearance by concentrating on your inward health as you age. He encouraged women to think about a nutritional face-lift before submitting to the scalpel. He urged his clientele to concentrate on nutrition and mental relaxation. He was way ahead of his time.

In *Mirror, Mirror On The Wall* Hauser talks about the importance of well-nourished tissues and how they affect each and every part of our bodies beginning with our face, which contains 55 muscles. A muscle is a muscle and whether that muscle is in your leg or face doesn't really matter. What matters is that each muscle is capable of great strength provided it is well-fed. Poor nutrition causes your muscles, all of them, to become slack. Well-fed muscles become firm and shapely rather than slack and flabby.[1]

A reliable plastic surgeon will tell you how long and how well a face-lift lasts depends not only on the skill of the surgeon but on how strong your facial muscles are. Even more damaging to facial contours is losing and gaining weight. When you are overweight, your facial muscles and tissues become soft and flabby, which in turn, stretches the skin. When this is followed by a quick reducing diet, the fat is all at once removed, and the face falls.

When you insist on dieting, don't be surprised when your muscles become starved for good protein, vitamins, and minerals. Dieting leaves nothing but fat and bloat, which destroys the most finely chiseled contours. Says Hauser, "If the candy-chewing, pastry-eating, soda pop-drinking ladies only knew what they are doing to their facial muscles, and through those muscles to their facial contours, they would lose no time in changing to the protein, high vitamin, high mineral diet that promotes health throughout your body, beginning with your face."[2]

Did I practice all Gaylord Hauser preached? In all fairness to the many readers who feel secretly ashamed, let me tell you that it took me years for these messages to sink in. Yes, I intuitively knew Hauser was right, but doing it was something else.

I knew that many of the people he talked about lived out their lives to a ripe old age and enjoyed the best of all worlds — they lived as long as possible without growing old.

Despite the lessons from Hauser and others, our country is facing an epidemic of ill health and obesity. But the wisdom of how to live long and healthily has been preserved even though it is not in common practice.

In keeping with my "best of all things" approach, I recommend reading *Successful Aging,* by John Rowe, M.D. and Robert Kahn, Ph.D. In their book the myths of aging are exposed using methods more scientifically advanced, but no more insightful and correct than Hauser's plan from forty years before. They debunk the myth that successful aging is largely determined by genetic inheritance.

Individual lifestyle choices GROW IN IMPORTANCE AND EFFECT as we age. In other words, by assuming responsibility for ourselves we can enjoy the physical and emotional health associated with youth — one of the central concepts of *Living Thin, Living Young*.

LIVING THIN WITHOUT COUNTING CALORIES — FOR THOSE PEOPLE WHO POSITIVELY, ABSOLUTELY REFUSE TO "THINK" CALORIES

Through all the years of teaching and learning about weight loss, I've seen it all — what works and what doesn't. I've seen trends and fads take off and burn out. Today, as we begin a new century, the problems of overweight and health risks are greater than ever. The More Things Change, The More They Stay The Same.

Unfortunately, there is more media coverage about obesity and diet advertising than ever. As our society becomes more addicted to TV and more dependent than ever on eating for entertainment, we wind up moving less and eating more. It's pathetic and sad, and it's enough to make me want to get a giant bucket of buttered popcorn and watch a triple feature just to get away from it all.

There are zones, pyramids, carb-loading, fat zapping, pill popping, wine-only, and beer-only programs designed to help you lose weight. The Living Thin way offers you an intelligent, educational solution for taking it off and keeping it off without giving up your favorite foods or having to engage in excessive exercise. It is simplicity plus!

Being educated means I am in charge. And being in charge means that I can have what I really want without gaining weight. What does "really want" really mean? It means now that I've been educated about the indisputable information about how my food choices and portion control affect my health and weight, I refuse to want or even desire, a lifestyle that includes a refrigerator or head that is filled with garbage. However, I also want to enjoy the privilege of knowing that a little garbage in either my head or my refrigerator won't spoil the deal.

In other words, I know that mindless eating is the major cause of my overweight, and that change takes time. However, I'm not in a hurry and, thank God, I don't have to be perfect.

When the message has been strongly and tightly planted in your head, and you have the strength to face the truth about the relationship between your weight loss efforts and your attitudes, you will be rewarded with the control you so desperately are seeking.

For those of you who are resisting, who are determined to Live Thin without counting calories, I am about to offer you an alternative method that will work if you work at it. There are books and programs devoted to losing weight easily by eating a high fat, high protein diet. Why does this method work?

The reason this method works is that eating proteins increases your metabolism by 30 percent, while eating carbohydrates increases your metabolism by only 6 percent. If you take two meals, one of veal and one of pasta, both of which provide the same calories (about 350), you will lose weight more quickly by eating the veal.

If it works, why am I opposed to this method? Simply because people I respect, Jane Brody (health reporter, *New York Times*), Dr. Jack Osman, and others tell me that this approach is unhealthy when practiced without moderation because of the stress it places on the kidneys.

However, after giving it much thought and by experimenting on myself and clients, I realized that I could apply this information to my Living Thin approach. It would be ideal for people who object to counting calories. But still, moderation and common sense are vital for its continued success.

Incidentally, the approach of high fat and high protein is not new. You may ask why has it not succeeded. Answer: for the same reason that the mindless counting of calories did not succeed. Any method that is rigid or boring and tedious is destined to fail.

By using the Living Thin approach, you cannot fail simply because of its simplicity and the absence of any "musts." There are no "musts" on this relaxed way of enjoying the journey.

Just to prove how old the issue of using high protein diets are, I want to tell you a story as related in a book by Gaylord Hauser about the use of a high protein, high fat style of weight loss. Hauser was a pioneer in natural health and a prophet of amazing insight.

In his book, *Gaylord Hauser's Treasury of Secrets* (published in 1951), he tells of an Englishman named Banning who, in 1851, made a marvelous discovery.[3]

At five feet, five inches and 200 pounds, he was made miserable by his bulkiness. When he reached 202 pounds and could no longer see his own feet, Banning became frantic and sought medical help. Doctor after doctor told him that he was eating too much and put him on very low-calorie diets. But he felt more miserable as his entire life seemed a hopeless battle against his excess layers of fat. Then a new misery descended on him. He started to lose his hearing.

Friends sent him to a fine ear surgeon who instead of ordering surgery, put Banning on a diet different from any he had ever followed. This time he ate the foods he liked best. In a year he had lost 50 pounds and 12 inches around the middle. And his hearing came back! He was so elated that he put his experiences in a booklet called, *Letter on Corpulence*. In it he reported what he ate and drank. Here was his daily fare:

BREAKFAST: 4 ounces of beef, mutton, kidney, liver, fish, bacon or cold meat (no pork), one slice of toast and a cup of tea without sugar.

LUNCHEON: 5 ounces of fish or meat (no pork), any kind of poultry, a choice of vegetable (no potato), one slice of toast, fruit for dessert and a glass of claret, sherry or Madeira wine (no beer or champagne).

TEA TIME: 2–3 ounces of fresh fruit, one slice of toast, and tea without sugar.

DINNER: Same as luncheon.

BEFORE RETIRING: If wanted, a glass of grog or a glass of sherry.

As you can see, the Banning regime was very high in calories. Thus, it could not have been the low-caloric intake that did the reducing; it was the low amount of carbohydrates. He stuck to his diet, omitted concentrated starches and sugars, kept his weight down to normal, and he lived a comfortable and long life. If your body is not equipped to handle carbohydrates, you can lose weight if you eliminate the beer and potatoes, cereal and grains, and severely limit the bread and pasta.

Basically, you can indulge in lean meats, seafood, yogurt, eggs, and salads IF YOU ARE DISCIPLINED ENOUGH TO DO WITHOUT THE STARCH.

Hauser stated that, "meat and fish proteins, eaten with a green salad tossed with a rich oil dressing, will pep up the metabolism and help you get rid of unwanted weight without going hungry." He identified the troublemakers as all cereals (with the exception of wheat germ), white sugar and white flour in all forms, cola drinks, all hydrogenated fats (with the exception of a tablespoon of sweet butter or nonhydrogenated margarine).

This alternative has been added to my Living Thin Program and is designed for people who are resistant to the concept of counting calories. However, you may want to combine the two approaches. Either way, it will work. Here are a few examples to get you started.

Breakfasts

1. 8 ounce glass of water. 1 slice of whole wheat toast with 1/2 pat butter. Two egg whites scrambled with tomatoes, onions, small bits of feta cheese. Black coffee or tea.

2. 8 ounce glass of water. Half a bagel with cream cheese, lox, and onions. Black coffee or tea.

3. 8 ounce glass of water. Two slices of French toast made with protein bread, dipped in batter. Recipe follows.

Batter: 1 Tbsp. butter, 1 Tbsp. canola oil, 1/4 cup cream, 1 egg, 1/2 tsp. vanilla extract, 1/2 tsp. maple extract, powdered cinnamon, and a dash of salt.

Heat butter and oil in frying pan. Place egg, cream, vanilla, and maple extracts in bowl and beat gently with whisk. Dip bread in bowl, then in frying pan until browned. Sprinkle cinnamon to taste.

Protein bread is higher in protein and lower in carbohydrates, thereby activating your metabolism as a protein would. Look for a high protein bread when you are using the Living Thin style of weight loss without counting calories.

Interchangeable Lunches and Dinner Suggestions

1. 8 ounce glass of water. Bowl of noncream-based soup. Huge tossed salad with water-packed tuna, shrimp or slices of turkey or chicken, tomatoes, assorted veggies, and low-cal dressing of your choice.

2. 8 ounce glass of water. Bowl of noncream-based soup. Broiled fish (grouper, salmon, mahimahi, swordfish). Tossed salad.

3. 8 ounces of water. Bowl of noncream-based soup. Crabmeat salad.

Snack and Dessert Choices

Plain yogurt with a spoonful of Polaner's jelly. Apple with 10 almonds (no salt or oil added). Guacamole with vegetable sticks. Custard. Cottage cheese and fruit. Cup of berries with sour cream or yogurt. Half a grapefruit. Biscotti and decaf coffee. 1/2 cup of low-fat hard-serve yogurt.

You may even treat yourself, on occasion, to a slice of angel food cake with fresh strawberries and some low-cal whipped cream.

Living Thin is absolutely the simplest way to gain control of our eating while gaining the freedom to enjoy the variety of foods that both please and satisfy us while we become mentally and physically healthier.

Because Living Thin advocates being in charge of your eating and making your own decisions, I recommend you experiment to find what works for you. My personal choice for intelligent, healthy, and permanent weight loss is counting calories (so simple it can be taught to a five-year-old.) I love the freedom it gives me. You will too.

The discipline of being moderate gives you the freedom to enjoy occasional excess — the essence of Living Thin.

THE BASICS: BECOMING AN ABSOLUTE SNOB ABOUT YOUR HEALTH

Daily Elimination: Weight Loss and Your Health

The good news about daily elimination is as follows:

1. You will lose weight more easily.
2. You will feel clearer in your head and your body.

3. You will be healthier physically and psychologically.

> Whoever has the responsibility holds the power.

In their book *Fit for Life II*, Harvey and Marilyn Diamond quote Dr. John H. Tilden, who discovered the phenomenon of toxemia in the early 1920s. (Toxemia is the process by which the body becomes diseased from failure to eliminate waste.) Tilden said, ". . . more often than not, what we call disease is nothing more than the body's own effort to cleanse itself of toxins."[4]

Several years ago, I recall developing an infection, probably a bacterial infection after a meal out. I was taken to the hospital where I enjoyed constant medical attention for six days. Every possible test that was available was given to me. After all the fussing, testing, and considerable expense of these procedures my doctor was convinced that all I needed was a thorough cleansing of my intestines, which I would have sworn were clear.

Following my cleansing, I left the hospital never to return. The solution was not complicated at all. I put myself on a higher fiber diet and never had the problem again.

A high fiber diet means including fresh vegetables, fruits, grains, and legumes (bean, lentils) in your daily meal plans. Every day, add one or two pieces of fruit; every day, one or two vegetables. Every day, add whole grain bread or cereal or as a side dish (pilaf, barley). Your protein needs will be met by eating a variety of these fibrous foods. You will get additional protein from dairy products, fish, and fowl.

Fiber, the nondigestible part of the food you eat, moves through your system like a broom to keep it clean and aids and promotes elimination of solid wastes.

Wondrous Water and its Magical Connection
to Weight Loss, Health, and Aging

"If I drink a lot of water, I'll be urinating all the time. That will be embarrassing."

"Coffee is made from water, that will be good enough."

"The only thing I like to do when I am not eating is drinking, and I will never be able to give up coffee and Coke. Anyway I drink diet sodas."

All through your life you have had to do things that were hard. Whether it was leaving your mother to go to kindergarten, leaving your hometown boyfriend to go to college, or dealing with personal setbacks such as moving to another city or losing a loved one. Now, in your efforts to lose weight permanently all I am asking you to give up are your excuses, ignorance, and misconceptions about your health that have led to your being overweight and feeling powerless to do anything about it.

Sure it would be terrific if you could break your giant cookie in half and all the calories would shake out of it. Or if a lemon cookie was a serving of fruit. Or if each portion of salad entitled you to the same number of portions of pie. Talk about pie in the sky! Real life requires that you get real. That's where Living Thin comes in. Living Thin is about education, health, and having the discipline to do the hard but satisfying things that give you self-respect and put you on the road to Living Thin.

Looking for a secret to successful weight loss? Well, here's one. Water. Ironic isn't it that we are constantly looking for easy answers, and the only ones that work are right under our noses. We continually ignore water for beverages that are brewed, bubbled, flavored, fermented, or pasteurized. As incredible as it may seem, water is quite possibly the single most important catalyst to losing weight and keeping it off.

Here are some startling, yet scientifically sound, facts about the benefits of water to weight loss:

- Water helps your body metabolize fat
- Water helps eliminate fluid retention
- Water helps you lose weight and keep it off

So, here you have another step in the educational process of becoming healthier and thinner. You can now throw away the diuretics and laxatives along with the appetite suppressants, while knowing that you never have to go back to them and are healthier for not doing so. The next time you have lunch with your best friend and she asks what you've done to make your skin and your figure look so great, say nothing. Make her go out and buy a copy of this book for herself!

Next to air, water is the element most necessary for survival. We've all heard that we can go weeks, or even months, without food, but only a few days without water before the system is traumatized. Short of that trauma, many people live in a dehydrated state, which is unhealthy because your insides are an internal sea. The body is actually two-thirds water, and every cell in your body depends on water to carry out its essential functions.

Water becomes even more important for someone trying to lose weight because you are likely to be eating a higher fiber diet, which increases your need for water. Whether you are on a high fiber diet or not, if you are not drinking enough water, you could end up with excess body fat, poor muscle tone, muscle soreness, or digestive complications.

Your body produces waste material as part of the digestion process. Daily elimination is so important because failing to do so turns you into a walking, talking toxic waste site. Water plays a central role in day-to-day elimination and cleansing as well as

> ## Water, water everywhere. DRINK UP! 8 glasses a day!

avoiding conditions related to auto-toxicity. Suffice it to say that keeping your insides clean is even more important than keeping your skin clean in terms of health. When deprived of adequate water, the body siphons what it needs from internal sources. The colon is one of those sources. The result? Constipation. When water is drunk by someone who is constipated, normal bowel function is usually restored.

Water plays a role in reducing fluid retention. When the body is deprived of water, it perceives this as a threat to survival and begins to hold on to every drop. This shows up as swollen feet, legs, and hands. The best way to overcome the problem of water retention is to give your body what it needs — plenty of water. If your water retention is related to excess salt intake, you need even more water to help your body dilute and excrete the sodium.

Water also helps to prevent the sagging of the skin and leaves skin clear and resilient. I was always delighted by how often I noticed the differences in people's skin while they were in my Living Thin classes. Within a few weeks of being on the program, I noticed the improvement. My experience tells me that any woman who wants to improve her skin tone and reduce facial wrinkles should understand how much more important water is on the inside than anything we could put on top of our skin. Many overweight people get away from skin wrinkles because the excess fat plumps up their skin. When you begin to lose weight and lose some of that fat, you will need to drink more water to provide the same plumping of the skin tissue.

Here is a blueprint for consuming 4–6 glasses of water per day (8 if you can handle it). And remember that when we talk about water; tea, coffee and sodas don't count. Experts agree that those drinks are not effective in regulating digestion and ridding the body of toxins.

So now you know what to do to make sure you're getting enough water. The gradual method is the best way to go. I began by putting a glass on my nightstand as a reminder to drink a glass first thing in the morning. Then I began playing mind games with myself. I imagined I was in a hospital with a nurse from the Little Shop of Horrors. In my scenario she told me I had to drink the entire glass or she was not going to leave the room. Down went the water. If you could have seen her, you'd realize how much easier it was to drink the water than to look at her.

You have my permission to be as devious or silly as you like as long as it works to get at least four glasses of water in you. You also need to be sure that the drinking takes place before and between meals. The reason for this is because water during meals dilutes digestive juices and inhibits full and speedy digestion of your food. It may be hard to keep up your resolve, but it will help to know that doing so will keep you feeling a little fuller all day long and lessen those ravenous feelings that make it so hard to stop nibbling.

To start, you do not have to carry a canteen around with you. Simply drinking four medium glasses of water will get you in the habit. After you establish the habit, you can slowly increase the size of your portion. Start with the glass you pick up off your nightstand in the morning. After drinking your first glass, just leave the glass by the sink in the kitchen. The next time you are there (to turn on the dishwasher or to rinse your breakfast dish), have another 8 oz. glass. It is that easy. Even if the next time you see that glass is in the evening, that's OK. Drink your next 8 oz. glass and you are up to three — with no change in your eating or drinking routine. In fact, drinking when you are not thirsty is best because thirst is not a good indicator of your fluid needs. If you wait until you are thirsty, you are already dehydrated.

Summary and instructions on the benefits of water for weight loss and good health: I want you to keep talking to yourself about the magic of water. Remind yourself: "I am going to drink my 4-6 glasses of water a day (or more) because it is going to help me lose weight easily, improve my daily elimination, keep me cleaner inside, and better looking outside. It will make my skin healthier and my kidneys will thank me too. Simply, water is one of the best things that could happen to any body, especially mine."

Sugar — Its Connection to Your Weight Loss and Your Health

The ordinary table sugar you eat every day will not only make you fat, but it could kill you!

"When I feel depressed or sad, the only thing that comforts me is a candy bar."

"I am not in control of my sweet tooth. And I don't want to be."

"Life is sweets. I will never be able to resist sweet food."

Living Rationally means "never saying never." You are a sugarholic. Do I ever know what that means! I was one. I beat it, but I still enjoy a sweet on occasion. And I still adore it, ON OCCASION. All the while I am in control of my weight. And you will be too. Just read on and listen to Sylvia.

This information about sugar is based on my own personal experiences, plus what I've learned by teaching clients with overweight problems for the past twenty years.

You can lose weight eating any kind of food including occasional cocktails providing it's calorie controlled. But that statement doesn't apply to sugar. Why? Because sugar causes your pancreas to spill insulin, and the insulin, in turn, stimulates your appetite. For some strange life-is-not-fair reason, this statement does not apply to people who are naturally slender. But since this book is not for them, just try not to die of envy and read on.

As long as you are trying to lose weight, you have absolutely no chance of succeeding as long as you insist on having sweets. Hold on now. Before you go running for a cookie, once you've reached goal weight, you can, on occasion, have a sweet provided you understand its connection to your weight control and to your health. I maintain that a little "poison" won't kill you, and my overall philosophy is one of moderation and common sense.

Two Things I've Learned About Sugar

After reading, teaching, and experimenting with myself and my students for twenty-five years, here are my conclusions:

1. Since sugar causes the pancreas to spill insulin, which in turn stimulates your appetite, sugar is an absolute no-no until you have begun to lose weight. Weight loss and even small amounts of sugar equal guaranteed failure. However, I have found that after a person reaches goal weight, he or she can indulge in a little "poison."

2. Because sugar is a chemical it is unhealthy for every part of my body. I happen to be concerned about my eyesight, which became a problem several years ago. I recall vividly asking Dr. Alan Gaby, a well-known medical nutritionist, if adding or subtracting any foods from my diet would help.

He assured me I was doing well but warned me against consuming sugar products. While I am aware of the dangers to my health and weight, being human, I do cheat on occasion. But sugar is a chemical. Don't ever forget it.

Sugar is that stuff that all overweights love — not only love, but are addicted to. Sugar is the single most important food/ habit challenge you will face. When your aversion to sugar matches your love for it, you will have it made.

White sugar or brown, honey or molasses, they all share one thing: you love them and they make you fat and unhealthy. Nobody could concoct a more effective conspiracy to make you fat, sick, and powerless than your relationship to sugar. It just so happens that the central character is YOU.

Sweets are what you turn to when you are feeling down, depressed, or upset. What you refuse to understand is that the stuff that makes you feel so good, the cookies, the brownies, the granola bars, and the pie is making you sick, tired and fat. As long as you fail to grasp this basic fact, you will waste your time, from now until the tomorrow that never comes, looking in vain for answers to your weight problem.

We've talked about sugar and weight gain. Now let's talk about sugar and health. Dr. John Yudkin was a distinguished British physician, biochemist, and researcher at London University from 1945–1954. He went on to do his work at the same university in the field of dietetics from 1954–1971. His pioneering studies of sugar (with people and animals) were recognized by medical journals throughout the world. Yudkin's work proves that the sugar we eat is directly related to the statistics we hear about diabetes, heart disease, and cancer. Dr. Yudkin's work raised a storm in the scientific world. But his book was really a call to the general public to recognize the crucial health hazards connected with refined sugar in the diet. Sadly, the controversy was confined to scientific and corporate interests alone, and the public never gained wide access to the information.

To quote Dr. Yudkin, ". . . if only a fraction of what is already known about the effects of sugar were to be revealed in relation to any other material used as a food additive, that material would promptly be banned."[5] Dr. Yudkin also describes in a delightfully British manner how the public, even the most educated and intelligent, protect themselves from unconventional views. The most common way is to view the messenger as a cranky sort who would rather rain on the parade — or in this case deprive us of our beloved sweets.

I know what goes on in the thought processes of people who want to lose weight (and especially in the minds of people who have tried and failed to lose weight over and again). You are likely reading about my Dr. Yudkin, thinking you've never heard of him and probably neither has your neighbor, co-worker, golf partner, or cab driver. Not only that, you're thinking that you don't need to heed Yudkin's warnings because research from other countries, even European ones, may not be up to American standards. And then there is the skepticism about me, the messenger. Well, I don't claim any academic or scientific credentials myself; however, I must respect the authority of those who do have those credentials and whose work is worthy of that respect, as should you and most other clear thinking people.

On the subject of sugar all agree — not only the people with whom I am in near total agreement, but also those with whom I am not. Dr. Yudkin's work no longer stands alone. In his book, *Dr. Atkins' Health Revolution*, Atkins cites Surgeon-Captain T. L. Cleave's book, *The Saccharine Disease*, as the "definitive essay" on sugar. Atkins continues, "Cleave shows example after example of societies in which the addition of sugar to the diet was the obvious starting point for the development of diabetes and of arteriosclerosis in the epidemic proportions typical for a Western nation."[6]

Dr. Lendon Smith, in writing the introduction to *Lick the Sugar Habit*, by Nancy Appleton, Ph.D., says it more simply yet. "We have heard the evils of sugar, from every writer in the world, except, of course, those from the sugar industry."[7] Actually, Appleton's book is a good resource for sugarholics or anyone interested in the ways that health is connected to body chemistry.

The word is out there about sugar and so is the resistance to it. But think for a moment, does Dr. Lendon Smith have anything personal to gain by identifying corporate sugar interests as self-serving deceivers of the public? Just look at what you can buy at the market, then judge for yourselves who it benefits to have so many sweets around all the time.

I call Dr. Yudkin "my Dr. Yudkin" because I have so much respect for his work and for his being free of the taint of corporate sugar's health-ignoring agenda. You see, sugar is BIG BUSINESS. Let's get that straight. Legislators in many countries often historically have taxed sugar to provide revenue just as they have often taxed tobacco and alcohol. And sugar resembles alcohol and tobacco in that it is a material for which people rapidly develop a craving and for which there is no physiological need.

As we discuss the connection between sugar and health, we see that "sugar" refers to a group of substances that have similar properties but are not identical. Fructose, lactose, maltose, sucrose, and glucose have made their way into our vocabularies and our diets. Simply put, fructose is fruit sugar, lactose is milk sugar, maltose is malt sugar, sucrose is ordinary table sugar, and glucose is a sugar found with other sugars in some fruits and vegetables. It's important to avoid being a purist on this subject because sugar has made its way into so many of our daily foods that leaving it out completely would leave you with a diet of bananas, peanuts, corn, and not much else. For instance, ketchup is likely to have sugar. But here is where not being a purist comes in; remember, eating a little ketchup won't make you fat.

No one understood the range of effects of sugar better than William Dufty. Dufty's story has an interesting background. He was a sugar addict himself, but kicked the habit under the influence of actress Gloria Swanson who was a natural foods advocate in her day. The result of Dufty's research is contained in his book *The Sugar Blues*. He concludes that sugar is a poison that has driven into our lives, uninvited at first by the health-ignorant profit motives of corporate sugar. He also shows the reader how to live better without sugar and offers recipes for delicious dishes — all sugar free. I just love the following quote from *The Sugar Blues*: "When a junkie dies, known or unknown, is it ever from 'metabolic complications'? Of course not. Heroin is a killer. Junkies die as a result of taking heroin. Even when a drunk dies, he dies of his sins. But when a person dies of 'sugar blues,' the mourners often serve sugar at the wake!"[8]

You see, your love affair with sugar may literally break your heart. It is also a fickle love. Though it temporarily frees you from a down mood, you wind up tired and fat. If you are sick and tired of being sick and tired, Living Thin is the answer.

My personal story is instructive because, like most, my addiction started innocently. I grew up during the depression. When my parents went into the grocery business, working at a store some distance from home, my mother would leave me enough money every day to go to the corner store for something to eat. And every day I would get a sugary confection. My favorite was custard pie with chocolate milk for lunch. I'd vary it from day to day by alternating plain custard pie with coconut custard pie. But I never failed to have the chocolate milk. And never failed to have a good time. I didn't realize it at the time, but I was in the early stages of a sugar addiction that contributed to my perennial weight problem.

When I invited Dr. Jack Osman to teach the early classes of Living Thin, he recommended that participants cut down or cut out sugar and sugary products. I learned a lot just by observing the class. The more I saw, the more I understood and became more convinced that the students couldn't get off the sugar simply because a doctor told them to. Nor could they permanently lose weight because Dr. Osman told them how.

At the time, there was little literature that could confirm what my instincts told me. I knew in my gut and in my brain that weight loss would not happen as long as sugar was prominent in the diets.

There was a nurse in the Living Thin class who explained the scientific details behind my intuitive understanding. When we eat sugar, the pancreas responds by spilling insulin into the blood, which in turn stimulates the appetite not just for sweets, but for all food.

Now I knew I was on to something. A real key. I refined my understanding through further experience. I learned that these events may not lead to obesity in every person, but they invariably do in people who are addicted to sugar. That is the bad news about sugar. The good news is that after you've broken the addictive cycle you can do as thin people do — have some sweets now and then.

There are two ways to give up your sugar addiction. One is to use artificial sweeteners with no calories, which may have health risks of their own, or to go cold turkey. The best way is to go cold turkey. That is the only way to overcome the obsession with sweet foods. It usually takes a few weeks and possibly a few headaches, but it is well worth it.

Before we get off the subject of sugar, I want to talk about changing your dietary patterns. The reason I want to go into this now, on the heels of my comments about sugar, is because I know how hard it is to give up long-held patterns, especially the one that includes sugar, because that is the hardest habit to break for so many overweight people. Sugar is the only "food" about which I make anything close to a hard and fast rule.

In order to make meaningful changes, each person has to be motivated enough to do whatever needs to be done. In this case, giving up sugar. If you are not ready to make that commitment, I suggest you put this aside until you are ready. Most of all, refuse to feel guilty about your decision.

I am giving you the tools for change. Using them is your choice.

NO MATTER WHAT DECISION YOU MAKE, OR HAVE MADE, YOU HAVE THE ABSOLUTE RIGHT TO YOUR CHOICES, WHATEVER THEY ARE.

However, if you are ready for change, it helps to see it as a challenge. And remember our old refrain, "I don't have to feel like doing it. I just have to do it."

So much for the pep talk. Remember, reading on its own doesn't count; what you do is what counts. It all starts with one step. Having been there myself, I know how loud the not-so-little voice inside your head will shout just as you are about to take that first step because the

> Sometimes you have to grit your teeth to do right.

very thought of giving up sweets terrifies you. You are happy to read for hours about how unhealthy sweets are, but it's when you put the book down that you find out if you've really learned anything.

Here's the blueprint for handling your sugar cravings. Start with the understanding that you are vulnerable when you are hungry, tired, or bored. So be on guard. Don't allow yourself to get hungry, and recognize when you are eating out of boredom or fatigue. I know and so do you — all too well — how easy it is to fall prey to the literally hundreds of opportunities for picking up a sweet.

You can continue to strengthen your resolve by watching people. When you see someone enjoying a big ice cream cone, take a look at their behind. That should give you some good aversion therapy to go along with your understanding about the connection between what people eat and the size of their . . . well, their physique. Here is that reminder again: having a sweet on occasion after you reach your goal weight won't mess you up!

If you must have a sweet: Try nonfat frozen yogurt as a sweet lifesaver. Several nonfat brands contain as few as 20 calories per ounce. But skip the toppings. They can mess you up. The savings in calories and the good sense of being restrained can be thrown into the trash if you go for the hot fudge topping. Frozen yogurt can be very satisfying and filling, making it a good trade-off.

If you want to find a sweetener to keep your fixation going, here is an option: health food stores carry a product called Stevia, which is technically an herb but acts like a very concentrated sweetener for coffee or tea. Or, Swiss Miss brand cocoa drink is made with artificial sweetener and will help you satisfy your craving without adding many calories. Also, Polaner's jelly is low in calories and can be used to sweeten a piece of toast.

You can, on your own, look for other items that will work as "helpers" in your efforts to get off the sweets-go-round.

Remember, you still need to count the calories in your sweet "rewards," and fat-free does not mean the same as low calorie.

Finally, let me try a scare tactic on you. It has worked for me. All the while you are reading and agreeing with me on the subject of sugar and sweets, a little voice is waiting for its moment to say, "Yeah, Sylvia is smart, and I can tell you are going along with her about all this stuff, but when you go into a restaurant, you just know you are going to think about ordering dessert in the form of cake, pie, or ice cream."

Well, here is how I took care of that little devil. Think about this: this is what happens when a fly lands on a piece of pie or cake. And you can be sure there are flies hanging around restaurants or they wouldn't have so many fly strips back in the kitchen. First, the fly vomits on the food to soften it up because it can't eat solid food. After vomiting, the fly stamps the vomit until it is liquefied. They are stamping in a few germs I'm sure, just for good measure. Then, when it's good and runny, they suck it all back up again. Probably dropping some excrement at the same time. When they've finished eating, it's your turn.

In summary, you can read the arguments about sugar until you are blue in the face but the most important part of this section is about your attitude.

> Love yourself
> unconditionally.

Let me be very emphatic here. While I am strenuously encouraging you to not eat white refined sugar while you are losing weight, I want you to avoid being a purist by skipping the ketchup. You need to understand that you must avoid thinking in such extreme terms.

The only forbidden food is the white refined sugar in the concentrations found in pies, cookies, and other similar goodies.

EXERCISE FOR PEOPLE
WHO REFUSE TO EXERCISE

For those of you involved with healthy activity patterns, you are excused from this section. For the rest of you, think if you've ever seen the following classified ad:

"Bicycles, stair climbers, treadmills. Barely used." (Some never used.)

"Will pay you to remove, along with a variety of exercise garments, barely used." (Some never used.)

The classified ads — the final resting place of so many good intentions to exercise, with someone willing to pay to get the remembrance out of their sight.

And now, physical fitness for all my DCs (difficult customers) who are involved with a series of excuses relieving them of the necessity of taking the first step toward healthy movement habits. I know that motivating a tired, flabby body to begin moving is tough. But it is not impossible. Trust me when I tell you that if you read and reread this portion on movement, you will begin moving more because I will provide you with a road map that is simply too simple to ignore. It will give you the

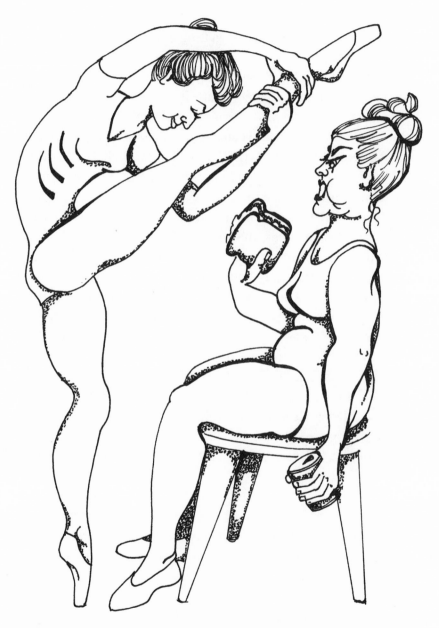

It's all a matter of priorities!

magic you are looking for — getting a tremendous return on a tiny investment.

In fact, if you are already eating sensibly you may not have to change your eating habits at all. In order for some of you to shed those extra pounds, exercise is ALL YOU MAY NEED. But for most of you who need a general overhaul of behavioral habits, remember: BY THE INCH IT'S A CINCH, BY THE YARD IT'S HARD. Remind yourself often of this trite but intelligent approach to change.

As far as the all-important start of a new behavior pattern is concerned, establishing the regular habit of exercise is even more important than the exercise itself. The benefits of merely getting started are vastly underrated. Who isn't better off exercising for even as little as five minutes as day, compared to someone who does not exercise at all? The minutes add up. Even at five minutes, it's hours per month. Once again, when you have the habit, the question is not whether or not you will exercise today, it is "for how long will I exercise today?"

One of my favorite writers on the subject of health is the late Dr. Jean Mayer. He said in one of his newsletters, that "combating overweight by diet alone is like fighting with one hand behind your back. Exercise is the other fist that enables us to deal the knockout punch."

For many men, women, and teenagers, moving more and eating less needs to become as routine as brushing your teeth. Study after study has shown that most people with weight problems do not eat too much. They simply move too little! Without some exercise, daily exercise, nearly all attempts to take it off and keep it off are doomed from the first fat-free, low calorie meal.

Unfortunately, the typical American sits in his car going to and from the workplace, sits at his or her desk or visits a nearby restaurant for lunch, goes back to work, or on to the bridge table or meeting table or theater seat. Lots of sitting . . . driving everywhere. Not much standing even. Even less moving.

Then it's back home for more sitting at dinner. Then it's in front of the television you go, where additional sitting is required. Until finally, the time has come to retire. Yes, you've become so exhausted from so much sitting that you have to lie down in bed!

Recently I drove a friend to the bank to get some money. She directed me to the Automatic Teller Machine. I had never used one, and my comment about never having used one, drew her chagrin. "Do you mean you park your car and go in the bank to get money?" she asked. I answered, "Not only that, I park as far away from the door as possible, take a short walk before I go in, and then take a short walk around the bank before I get back to my car." She was flabbergasted.

She is also forty pounds overweight and has a host of health problems connected to her being overweight, not the least of which is arthritis. She is part of a society that increasingly makes it possible to avoid even the simplest form of movement/exercise — walking. You don't even have to walk across the room to change the television channel.

This all happens while the television reports about the decline in our health that everyone laments and feels powerless to stop. Do you see the problem here? There is an epidemic, and instead of doing anything about it, we all complain about it. Sound familiar? *"I want to lose weight and be healthy, but it's too hard."*

The solution is to start doing 3–5 minutes of movement exercise every day the Living Thin way. Be forewarned, I've removed all your excuses.

Not only does this nonactive lifestyle promote overweight with big tummies and big behinds, but it also encourages a host of ailments that could, with daily exercise, be avoided. Regular movement with the lowest levels of exertion will reset your body's thermostat. You can actually lower your metabolic set point for calorie burning during nonexercise periods with minimal amounts of exercise! Yes, I said MINIMAL!

Sedentary living is like being sentenced by a judge to a guaranteed life of failing to win the battle of the bulge. By dictate of this sentence you will experience periods of self-denial (dieting), followed by guilt when self-denial gives way to self-indulgence (undisciplined bingeing and eventual loss of portion control).

The following unfortunate scenario affects the thinking and behavior of overweights. It is unfortunate because it gives rise to greater discouragement for those struggling to simply begin exercising. You have struggled to lose 10–20 pounds, your clothes don't fit, and you hate it. You feel motivated to begin an exercise program and grab a magazine that has an article on exercise and weight loss. The article says you will need to walk four miles to burn the calories contained in a single slice of pie. I know what your reaction is. You are saying, "I know I will not walk four miles. I feel defeated and sad. I am going to grab a bag of cookies and sit in front of the TV."

A much better formula for success is to first understand that daily exercise revs up your body's engine so that your body continues to use extra calories for up to 15 hours after you stop exercising. That means that if you exercise for as little as 3–5 minutes in the morning and the evening, you get a calorie burning bonus all day long and all night long even when you are sleeping and even if your body's metabolism is on the slow side. Yes, exercise can boost your metabolism permanently by 20–30 percent once your exercise habit gradually reaches above your starter level.

And that ain't all! Here is a super fact reported by the eminent health reporter for *The New York Times*, Jane Brody. According to studies done at Cornell University, exercise done 2–3 hours following a meal uses up more calories than the same exercise done on an empty stomach! This is because exercise turns up the body's thermostat when it follows a meal (by 2–3 hours) than on an empty stomach. This great news means you can eat more and weigh less if you are just willing to pick up your feet and take a short walk, jog in place on the carpet or on a trampoline, or do the bicycle while lying on the floor with your legs up in the air. Any movement that is vigorous will do to get started if done for even as little as 3–5 minutes. Vigorous means done without interruption and at a level that raises your heart rate. Dawdling down the block and stopping to talk to the neighbors won't cut it.

Here are other fringe benefits you get from exercising regularly, no matter how little:

You will lose body fat and replace it with lean muscle tissue. Pound for pound, the more muscle tissue you develop, the less body fat you have.

The more motivated you are to continue this pattern of movement the healthier you will become, the more energy you will have to help cope with and overcome some of the problems associated with the aging process. You can only win the game of health when you decide to move more, so get a move on!

Another word about the upside of developing muscle tissue: it takes up less room than the same amount of fat. That means you will look thinner even if you haven't lost an ounce. The mirror doesn't lie!

Losing weight on a low calorie diet that is not accompanied by a daily exercise program is a much slower process than losing while you do a modest amount of daily exercise.

A 500 calorie deficit in your daily diet will add up to one pound of body fat lost in a week. A low calorie diet may allow you to lose 3–5 pounds of water and muscle during your first week or two. But subsequent weeks of calorie counting without exercise will not produce the same loss of muscle and water.

As a result, many become discouraged and quit at this point. You've probably been there. I certainly have seen and felt it myself. A much better approach for your health and for permanent loss is to lose primarily fat in the first place. And the only way to do so is by exercise. The simple reason is that exercise uses body fat as its main source for energy.

You may not see that initial, rapid (but short-lived) rate of loss, but what you do lose is exactly what you want to lose most — fat, not muscle or water. Your loss will be slow but steady, and if you continue to exercise, you can realistically picture yourself being slender forever.

Statistics tell us that in most cases the faster people lose weight, the more likely they are to regain it. Slow loss is the secret. Be the tortoise, not the hare.

There are other exciting benefits of developing the habit of moving more and sitting less. When you move more and sit less, the exercise suppresses your appetite. Who needs the pills and potions? And because exercise is a natural relaxant, it reduces the chances of your eating for the wrong reasons, namely, boredom, depression, anger, etc. Those good feelings that are produced by exercise are most likely the result of the body's secretion of a natural tranquilizing chemical, beta-endorphin. It is released in the brain in response to exercise. This chemical is the body's equivalent of Valium or morphine. However, beta-endorphin lacks the expense and adverse side effects associated with drugs.

I recall vividly telling my students, "If you insist on feeling depressed, you will have to wait until you've had your walk or completed your 5–10 minute exercise for the morning or evening."

Scientists have demonstrated that it is almost impossible to feel depressed while you are in motion. (This recommendation about postponing your depression is for mature people only. The rest of you can just go ahead and pout.)

What Exactly Do I Need to Do to Get Started?

At the time I was beginning my first few Living Thin classes, I naturally read every book printed on the subject of exercise and weight loss. I was amused and annoyed when all the so-called experts insisted on the importance of a minimum of 20 minutes of exercise at a time. For the Difficult Customer who never exercises, who is not ashamed to let other people do the work of simply opening a door or fetching a glass of water for them, doing 20 minutes of exercise times a week is ludicrous.

For this reason I began asking my students to think of any vigorous activity they could do for 3–5 minutes (180–300 seconds) at home. They could choose jogging in place on a rug or trampoline or lying on their backs with their legs up doing "the bicycle" as I do. Whatever they chose, I insisted that they deny themselves the right to leave the house until they had completed a 3–5 minute period of brisk movement. Just that much movement revs up the body's motor, begins burning calories more efficiently, provides extra energy, and best of all, begins the habit. THE HABIT IS MORE IMPORTANT THAN THE DURATION. The time will follow naturally.

The failure to exercise is NOT based on a failure to recognize its benefits. IT IS FROM UNWILLINGNESS TO MAKE TIME. Once you decide to develop a new pattern of behavior, then you never have to face the crisis over whether or not you have the time to exercise. The decision is a done deal.

To get started and to keep going, look hard and think hard about fitting some basic physical movements into places where now there is none.

How Can I Motivate Myself to Begin Moving More and Sitting Less?

You may be saying to yourself, "I know how great the benefits are but my motivation has never been strong enough to keep up the exercise habit." I know where you are. You are still inactive and aren't even in the game yet.

I must repeat the old refrain: "I DON'T HAVE TO FEEL LIKE EXERCISING. I JUST HAVE TO EXERCISE. AND GUESS WHAT? SOON I WILL FEEL SO MUCH BETTER, I WILL BE SEARCHING FOR OPPORTUNITIES TO INCREASE MY TIME SPENT EXERCISING."

Starter Tips — Mental Jogging

The issue of time is always part of beginning a new habit. It's important to point out how much time you will find if you wind up with arthritis, osteoporosis, or angina. I know, I've seen it happen and I've been there myself.

Remember, the benefits you derive from daily exercise (even if it's minimal) are immediate. These short range pluses are followed by the long term, highest-yield benefits — a healthy life that you are in charge of.

The mental jogging I am referring to involves reviewing the information in this book on self-talk. Also remind yourself often that you cannot afford the luxury of ignoring the obligation you have to yourself for daily exercise and to be as healthy as you can. The choice is yours. If that sounds like bad news to you, the good news is that it can be a little as ten minutes, twice a day. Even at this low rate your body will respond in a variety of healthy ways.

Remember, it's not how long you exercise but how consistently you exercise. It must become a habit whether it is one that you enjoy every minute of or not. The issue of time will resolve itself by starting with a short duration and the available time will automatically increase once you have established the habit of movement.

Starting Tips — Find Your Own Ways

Simply park farther away from your destination. If you aren't an exerciser, I guarantee that when you climb a flight of stairs instead of taking the elevator, your heart will be beating just like it would if you were in a gym or at a spa. Imagine, with nothing more than a flight of stairs, the possibility of gaining improved health opens before your eyes and under your feet. Just think "MOVEMENT."

And think "SOCIAL." Invite a friend to walk with you or step with you. You don't need a partner, however. You can even dance alone to your favorite CD or radio station. What makes it all work is your forcing yourself to become involved in movement activities. Your expectations are important too. Don't expect to love your activity immediately. In due time you will be *so* glad that you've made it a part of your life.

A Case Study

My friend Susan suddenly began experiencing severe arthritis pain in her ankles and knees. I was amazed at how much time she devoted to thinking about, planning around, and complaining about her situation.

She was being treated by a nationally recognized specialist who was taking painfully long in coming up with the correct combination of anti-inflammatory drugs and steroids to give her enough relief to permit her to travel to see her children and grandchildren.

Susan was in pain, suffering from depression, and confused over how she was going to continue the everyday activities to which she was accustomed.

Had she found the time to develop a healthy lifestyle — meaning a combination of good food choices and including minimal daily movement — many experts agree that even if she had not been able to avoid the arthritis entirely, she would be likely to have far less severe symptoms.

Do you truly believe there will ever be a time when time is not of major importance to your life? Of course not! By simply forcing yourself to incorporate anywhere from 3–12 minutes of exercise movement, you will be buying the best insurance policy you can have — the one that is cheap and gives you more health. In slightly longer than it takes to brush your teeth, you can begin a habit (that's all brushing your teeth is) that will make you look and feel better and healthier.

To free yourself from the confusion about exercise and health, I offer a few simple guidelines:

No more excuses. They are unacceptable and take you down a blind alley. If you keep finding reasons for not doing what you know you should do, reread my approach: No more than 10 minutes a day, EVERY DAY. The habit is more important than the length of time. Increasing the time is a simple matter. Developing the habit is the issue.

Become an observer. When you hear yourself finding reasons for avoiding doing any exercise, refuse to accept it. Just as you would if a little voice inside told you to skip brushing your teeth. Also, try taking a trip to a few facilities such as a retirement/nursing community. If you are fortunate and smart, you may avoid being in one of them.

Think hard. Think about some of the illnesses that could have been avoided in part or entirely had these incapacitated people done their homework and simply done some modest exercise every day of their lives.

Thank your lucky stars. Consider your fortune to have all the body parts you need and that you can use them.

Don't miss your chances. If, for example, you need to leave home at 6 a.m. to catch a plane, allow 3 minutes for an exercise activity. Even if you are scheduled for an operation at the hospital or at the doctor's office, do some exercise first. Even after an operation, the sooner you can safely begin moving again, the faster you will heal.

It must be said that if you have a medical problem, your physician should be consulted. But while we are talking about consulting your doctor, ask him or her to confirm what I am telling you: that even moderate exercise works to lower the risks of heart disease and stroke by lowering serum cholesterol levels and by improving the ability of the heart to pump blood with less effort. See if your physician has a comment on how exercise strengthens your bones by preventing the loss of calcium as we age and, as long as exercise is not overdone, helps keep joints mobile, which wards off the crippling effects of arthritis.

If your doctor has been doing his or her homework, you can learn more about improving the quality of your sleep and your moods from exercise. If your doctor seems unfamiliar with these ideas, you may want to shop around for someone new with whom to consult even if you keep your current doctor. Many doctors now insist on including an exercise program for patients suffering from extreme mood swings, anxiety, frustration, guilt, and even depression. Are you aware of the studies that show people who exercise daily enjoy better sex lives — both in quality and quantity! (However, be wary about devoting too much time to exercising, you may wind up with too little time for sex!)

So there you have it. Healthy and permanent weight loss includes exercise of some kind, not much, every day. It can start with as little as swinging your arms forward and backward and alternately tapping your toes and heels and wiggling your fingers. Do it twice daily and three times on Sunday.

Find ways to move more and sit less. Never forget for a moment that a major reason you are overweight is simply because you move too little.

> **Your Heart Needs Exercise.**

Exercising involves much more than just your waistline. It affects your health and how you age.

Case Study

My friend Roz is a splendid example of the benefits that simple movement can make to your immediate health. Roz is not a kid anymore, and she has some health problems. But what an attitude! She suddenly found that she couldn't walk very much without torturous pain in her legs. She listened to a lecture at a neighborhood hospital where she was directed to develop an exercise program that would help with her problem. Roz learned quickly and put the recommendation into action just as quickly. And guess what? She is back to her usual, noncomplaining, busy lifestyle.

Although Roz is in her 80s, she simply has never had time for illness. What was the secret to her recovery? Simple. Every day she would stand and do a slow "jig." To get her circulation going and regain her freedom to walk without pain, she'd rise up on her toes, then down on the heel and then do the same on the other foot. She does it every day and has never had to lie in bed waiting for someone to come along and "do it" for her.

I was inspired by Roz's story. I also know that after you put this book down you may find an article that says, "Walking will never get you fit." Well, I have books on my shelf that say, "Walking provides top-notch aerobic training." If you do nothing but walk for exercise, you will have it made.

Both your article and my book cite scientific research to support the views. Because of the conflicting, confusing, and often misleading information to which we are subjected, using your own common sense is more vital than ever. THINK. Does it make sense to say walking is not beneficial?

Then there are publications that urge you to check out the information you read. In other words, to become an expert about the so-called experts. The time this would take could be used for exercise! I fail to understand how people who use time for an excuse for avoiding exercise could find the time to check out the experts.

Let's concentrate on old-fashioned common sense. Listen to my suggestions for beginners and take it from there. It's not complicated. It's painfully simple. It does not require any machinery or special shoes or clothing. But it WORKS.

If you insist on continuing to be a Difficult Customer and refuse to get started, I'd urge you to set aside all your efforts to lose weight until another time when you are thinking more clearly. But remember, in the future you will still be confused about conflicting information in the media about health and exercise, you still won't feel like exercising, you still won't be in the habit, and you will still have to deal with the garbage in your head and on your plate.

You do have the right to decide now is not the time, but there is no time like the present. You are only 200 seconds or so from having completed the first step. Forget yesterday. Yesterday is gone. But prepare for tomorrow, whatever your age is at this moment, and feel better today.

Living Thin is based on the three elements required for healthy, permanent weight loss: attitude training, health education, and exercise. I've learned that there is a lot of valuable information that hasn't been combined in simple, useful ways for people with a weight problem. What I have done is to bring the information together to provide a blueprint for controlling your efforts to lose weight healthily and permanently.

Please read what I am about to tell you carefully and slowly. Remember it so that you can remind yourself of its importance:

> It is natural for you to be tempted to reject a new idea when you hear it: namely, that as little as five minutes of exercise daily will make a big difference to your physical fitness. All too often the first thing people do with a new idea is to measure it against an old one. And if the new idea conflicts with the old one, the new one will be rejected.

After so many years of teaching my Living Thin lifestyle and so many successful students, I know these ideas are tried and true. You have nothing to lose but weight and so much to gain in the realm of fitness.

SUMMARY

This chapter is all about an intelligent solution to permanent and healthy weight loss. You've already experienced the only other choice — namely victimizing yourself by accepting choices others are making for you. Living Thin is about educating you so you can make your own choices about food and portions. Only until, and unless, you can make your own choices that are compatible with your lifestyle and eating tastes, can the program be permanent.

While I was writing this portion of the book, I was working with Esther who for years had resisted and refused to count calories. During the very first week of doing so, however, she told me that for the first time she knew she was "in charge."

How does counting calories put you in charge? In the same way as knowing how much you can afford for anything you desire puts you in charge. Only when you are making the choices will it last. However, for those hardheads among you, I am saying to read the portion about not counting calories and that will work for you too, IF YOU CAN HANDLE IT. This program is all about choices. It is completely up to you.

I have included suggested Living Thin meal plans on the following pages to give you an idea of some well-balanced, nutritious menu selections. Do not view these as rigid menus, though, that you must follow to Live Thin. These are merely my interpretation of Living Thin — what works for me. Please (and I can't stress this enough) be Ready, Willing, and Able to devise your own interpretation of Living Thin — to select foods you like, that are nutritious and convenient. Because Living Thin is, above all, about you being in charge.

Everyone wants to live as long as possible and never grow old. Data coming out tell us that life span and quality of life are indeed determined largely by your ongoing lifestyle choices. Age is not an enemy; illness is.

Aging disgracefully versus aging gracefully is not about years, it about the process that determines whether your body can continue to restore itself in the 20–30 years beyond what is now considered normal life expectancy. This is the difference between ugly aging and happy aging, regardless of your chronological age.

The best way to meet this challenge is to develop a lifestyle that will let you be young from the inside out — by exercising, boosting your immune system, becoming educated about nutrition, breathing fresh air, and controlling your stress. And most of all, controlling your weight.

MEAL PLANS FOR LIVING THIN

BREAKFASTS
200 to 250 calories

Have coffee or tea as you wish. We recommend whole wheat bread, but feel free to use rye, etc.

#1

8 oz. water	0
1/2 c. oatmeal	70
1/2 c. skim milk	40
1 banana	100
TOTAL:	210 calories

#2

8 oz. water	0
1 orange	60
1 poached egg	80
(Sprinkle with black pepper & chives or other herb)	
1 slice whole wheat toast	60
1/2 pat butter	17
(Pat of butter is 1 inch square and 1/3 inch thick . . . 35)	
1 broiled tomato	0
TOTAL:	217 calories

#3

8 oz. water	0
1 c. strawberries *or*	
1/2 c. blueberries *or* small apple	50
1/2 c. low fat cottage cheese	
sprinkled with cinnamon	100
2 rice cakes	60
TOTAL:	210 calories

#4

8 oz. water	0
1/2 grapefruit	40
1 Nabisco Shredded Wheat biscuit	90
3/4 c. skim milk (Try warming milk	
and sprinkle cereal with cinnamon)	60
TOTAL:	190 calories

#5

8 oz. water	0
1/4 cantaloupe	30
1/2 wheat bagel	80
with sliced tomato and 1 oz.	
part-skim mozzarella cheese	
(Place in broiler until cheese melts)	70
TOTAL:	180 calories

#6

8 oz. water	0
1 banana	100
1 slice whole wheat toast	60
spread with 1/4 c. low fat cottage	
cheese and top with cinnamon	50
TOTAL:	210 calories

#7

8 oz. water	0
1 orange	60
1 oz. All-Bran	70
1/2 c. skim milk	40
1/2 c. strawberries	25
TOTAL:	195 calories

Weekend options:

Omelet: 1 egg with 1/4 c. skim milk, fry in PAM, season with black pepper and chives or other herbs. 1 slice whole wheat toast with 1/2 pat butter.

TOTAL: 180 calories

French toast: Soak 2 slices whole wheat bread in a mixture of 1 beaten egg, 1/4 c. skim milk, 1/2 tsp. vanilla extract and dash of nutmeg. Fry in PAM. Spread with 2 tsp. Polaner fruit spread.

TOTAL: 224 calories

LUNCHES
250 to 320 calories

Have coffee or tea as you wish. With all of these lunches add as many "free" vegetables as you like, i.e., raw carrots, celery, red, yellow and green peppers, turnips, broccoli, cauliflower, cucumber, etc. or have a large bowl of "free" soup. (Take it with you in a thermos.)

#1

8 oz. water	0
3½ oz. can salmon	135
onions, cucumber, and dill if desired	0
lettuce and tomato	0
1/2 wheat bagel, toasted	80
with 1/2 pat butter	17
TOTAL:	232 calories

#2

8 oz. water	0
sandwich w/ 2 slices whole wheat toast	120
4 oz. turkey breast	180
lettuce, tomato and whisper of mayo	0
TOTAL:	300 calories

#3

8 oz. water	0
sandwich w/ 2 slices whole wheat toast	120
4 oz. chicken breast	200
lettuce, tomato and whisper of mayo	0
TOTAL:	320 calories

#4

8 oz. water	0
l large wheat pita pocket filled with tomato, onion, spinach or lettuce, cucumber, green pepper and 1/2 oz. crumbled feta cheese. Sprinkle with pepper and herbs.	215
	TOTAL: 215 calories

#5

8 oz. water	0
1 small wheat pita pocket filled with a 3½ oz. can of water-packed tuna, celery, onion, lettuce and a whisper of mayo	210
	TOTAL: 210 calories

#6

8 oz. water	0
1 slice whole wheat bread spread with Dijon mustard	60
1 oz. provolone cheese	100
sliced tomato, mushroom, onion, sprouts and lettuce	0
(Pile it all on and make a "Dagwood")	
small apple	50
	TOTAL: 210 calories

#7

8 oz. water	0
vegetable bowl: add any combination	
of "free" vegetables, e.g., cauliflower,	
broccoli, celery, romaine lettuce, carrots,	
red and green peppers, cucumber, etc.	0
1 oz. feta cheese	75
low-cal dressing	20
2 slices whole wheat bread	120
1 pat butter	35
TOTAL:	250 calories

Weekend options:

"Free" vegetable soup (recipe on page 187). Vegetable Melt: Steam variety of vegetables: cauliflower, broccoli, carrots. Sauté onions and mushrooms in Pam. Toast 2 slices of whole wheat bread, put on whisper of mayo. Place steamed and sautéed vegetables on top of toast. Slice tomatoes and place on top of vegetables. Top with 2 slices part skim mozzarella cheese and place in oven until cheese is melted.

Baked potato, topped with black pepper and Dijon mustard . . . or nonfat plain yogurt, chives and parmesan cheese — or 1/4 pat butter   TOTAL: 120 calories

Baked potato with poached egg on top. TOTAL: 120 calories

Baked potato with steamed vegetables and parmesan cheese on top.   TOTAL: 120 calories

DINNERS
320 to 500 calories

Have coffee or tea as you wish.

#1

8 oz. water	0
spinach and red onion salad	0
1 Tbsp. low-cal salad dressing	20
3 oz. baked turkey breast	135
1/2 large sweet potato	80
pat of butter	35
string beans	0
broiled tomato	0
small baked apple	50
TOTAL:	320 calories

(Bake or microwave sweet potato & apple together).

#2

8 oz. water	0
1-egg cheese omelet:	
1 egg (+ 2nd egg white, if desired)	80
1 oz. part skim mozzarella cheese	70
1/2 c. skim milk	40
sauté in 1/2 pat of butter	20
sauté onion, green pepper, garlic and mushroom in Pam	0
1 wheat toast w/ 1/2 pat butter	80
1/2 frozen banana	50
TOTAL:	340 calories

#3

8 oz. water	0
romaine lettuce and carrot salad	0
1 Tbsp. low-cal salad dressing	20
4 oz. broiled scallops	
(Top with lemon juice and black pepper).	180
1/2 c. white rice, cooked	110
asparagus	0
broiled tomato	0
1/2 c. strawberries	25
TOTAL:	335 calories

#4

8 oz. water	0
romaine lettuce with sprouts	0
1 Tbsp. low-cal salad dressing	20
3 oz. baked or broiled half chicken breast	
(Marinate in orange juice, low-sodium	
soy sauce and crushed garlic)	150
1 med. baked potato	100
1/2 pat butter	20
broccoli	0
cauliflower	0
1 c. watermelon pieces	40
TOTAL:	330 calories

#5

8 oz. water	0
lettuce and sliced tomato	0
1 Tbsp. low-cal salad dressing	20
1½ c. pasta, cooked	275
topping of sautéed tomato, onion,	
garlic, green pepper, and snow peas	0
in 1/2 pat butter	20
fresh peach	35
TOTAL:	350 calories

#6

8 oz. water	0
1 c. "free" vegetable soup	0
3 oz. broiled hamburger patty	230
1 corn on the cob	85
with 1/2 pat butter	20
asparagus	0
sliced tomatoes	0
1 c. unsweetened applesauce	100
sprinkled with nutmeg	0
TOTAL:	435 calories

#7

8 oz. water	0
4 oz. tomato juice	30
3 oz. broiled orange roughy	80
(or other non-oily fish) . . . top with lemon juice, herbs, and black pepper)	
1/2 c. white rice, cooked	110
carrots	0
mushrooms	0
1/2 cantaloupe	95
TOTAL:	315 calories

#8

8 oz. water	0
romaine lettuce with cucumber	0
1 Tbsp. low-cal salad dressing	20
1 5-oz. veal chop	260
1 medium baked potato	100
with 1/2 pat butter	17
broiled tomato	0
string beans	0
pear	100
TOTAL:	497 calories

RECIPES:

Homemade dips/spreads

Mustard-mayo: Combine 2 Tbsp. Dijon mustard, 1/2 c. low fat mayo. 35 calories per Tbsp.

Mustard Yogurt: Combine 1/2 c. Dijon mustard with 1/2 c. plain yogurt. 20 Calories per Tbsp.

"Free" Vegetable Soup

1 med. sized cabbage, sliced
1 large onion, sliced
4 stalks celery, chopped
4 carrots, sliced
1 24 oz. can Italian plum tomatoes
1 8 oz. can tomato sauce
2 tsp. thyme
Fresh minced garlic (to taste)
Freshly ground black pepper
3 dashes red pepper flakes (optional)

Cover with water, bring to a boil and simmer until vegetables are tender (40–60 minutes). Add other "free" vegetables if you like. Freezes well. Serve with parmesan cheese sprinkled on top.

Veal Chop

Mix 1 tsp. Worcestershire sauce, 1/8 tsp. garlic powder, 1 Tbsp. Dijon mustard and 1 tsp. vegetable oil together. Spread half of mixture on one side of chop. Broil 3 inches from heat for 5–7 minutes, until brown. Turn chop and spread with remaining mixture. Broil 5 minutes or until done to taste.

Chapter 6

Living Thin On The Run

Planning, Eating on the Run, Recipes and More...

A Blueprint for Planning

The key to change is PLANNING. I know you don't want to hear this. You don't want to take the time. It's much easier to follow a plan made by someone else. Unfortunately, it doesn't work. The only plan that works is YOUR plan. If it has your name attached to it, your chances for following it are raised considerably. With someone else's plans, as with people you don't like, you will go to great lengths to avoid them.

For permanent and healthy weight loss you want to examine your eating, activity, and relationship patterns. Then decide what needs fixing. The intelligent solution means finding a way of eating, exercising and, above all, of handling daily stress that evolves into lifestyle patterns that are designed for YOU ALONE. That's why it works.

To begin, examine your attitudes. Accept that your negative feelings — depression, anxiety, anger, general upsettedness — do not come from a specific situation but from the thoughts you choose to tell yourself about a situation.

> If you don't know where you're going, you might wind up somewhere else.
>
> Yogi Berra

To fix an attitude, you need first to identify the head talk that is causing the feeling (go back to Chapter 2 for specific information).

Avoid changing too much too soon. If you identify several issues you want to work on, go even more slowly, so that you won't become overwhelmed and give up. You might begin by selecting one or more habits on the "Habit List" that is included in this section: for example, eating while on the run. We are all in a hurry these days. That's not likely to change. You can eat on the run IF IT'S PLANNED! Simply plan what you are going to eat when you are on the run.

You might decide to carry fruit with you and some of the health bars I'll show you how to make at home. That will do it for you if you are on the go constantly. Don't forget to put it on your eating chart, though. That is where your plans are translated into a matter of record.

For exercise, if you are not involved in movement now, nothing, repeat NOTHING, is stopping you from going up and down a flight of stairs (yours or someone else's) several times a day.

The best part of making a plan is that once you convince yourself of the value of planning, then doing it becomes quite easy. Planning is all about YOU. It gives you the joy of being in charge when you are feeling uptight, worried, or hassled about being overweight; things which very often happen simply because you have no plan! It is the absence of having a plan that leaves you lost and feeling powerless.

Planning without doing doesn't count! One of my students told me, "I've decided to become a planner. Now I'm finding that I spend a lot of time planning. But guess what? Nothing much is happening. I make plans, then I become so tired, so bored with devoting so much time to the planning part that I find myself walking away from the 'doing' part."

If this is in your head, just listen to what you are saying. You're saying you've gone from 0 MPH to 90 MPH, and instead of having no plan at all, you are now into too much planning. The lesson is LESS TIME WITH THE PLANNING AND MORE TIME WITH THE ACTION PART. The key as always is moderation and common sense (M & C, what this whole book is about!). Nothing will change until you take action, but planning comes first. Just don't stop when the plan is made; take the next step.

Planning That Works

1. TALK ABOUT YOUR PLAN. Talk to any and everyone who will listen. Each time you tell someone else what you plan to do you are reinforcing your priority.

2. SET REALISTIC GOALS. Be sure your food planning includes foods you will enjoy. You don't want to feel deprived or hungry — ever. By seeing to your enjoyment, you avoid setting yourself up for failure. Be sure to include some choices you love, EVERYDAY. It's all about moderation and common sense, NOT ABOUT DEPRIVATION.

3. REFUSE TO BECOME INFLEXIBLE. When you insist on being inflexible, you are setting yourself up for guilt feelings when you goof. Give yourself a break. RELAX.

Perfectionism will leave you in a state of constant stress. It also is clear by now that stress drives you to overeat.

4. PLAN FOR THE UNPLANNED. Have a backup plan. For instance, if you exercise by walking around the block, have a "plan B" in place if the weather becomes too severe. If you go to a gym and your instructor gets married and goes on a honeymoon, you can substitute exercise at the gym by climbing five flights of stairs in your apartment building twice a day or jog in place while you watch TV.

5. REFUSE TO BECOME UPSET IF YOU CAN ONLY HAVE HALF A PLAN. Half a plan is much better than no plan. It means you are not giving up on planning.

6. PLAN TO PLAN. Make planning a priority. Develop the habit of thinking about how you want each day to develop.

Making unexpected changes is easy when you have a plan. Instead of wasting time agonizing over a change, simply review your plan and use your time to make the adjustment. Planning helps you to know where your priorities lie.

Suppose you are scheduled to go out for dinner, but for a variety of reasons (a sudden snowstorm or lack of transportation), you cannot leave the house. You have food in the house that will allow you to switch your plans suddenly and still be moderately satisfied and not involve any weight gain. You make half a dish of ratatouille and have a portion of fruit with custard for dessert and you've got it made.

Let's examine the fringe benefit of making a plan for yourself rather than having someone else make it for you.

The success of your plan is based on achieving the goals you've set for yourself. Whenever you feel your old resistance to planning, force yourself to think of the consequences. When you say, "To heck with planning. Let the chips fall where they may," ask yourself where they are most likely to fall.

Without a plan your old habits will surface. The noshing and nibbling, the very same habits that produced the problem, will never go away if you fail to plan.

Is there a guarantee that you will never return to old habits? Of course not. But you will begin to understand and to accept that your problems have more to do with a rotten attitude than it had to do with food. Somewhere along the way you failed to learn how to discipline yourself, the discipline that comes from creating a plan. The ideal person to create the plan is YOU. When the planning comes from you, it increases the probability of success.

Planning sets you free from having to make constant decisions. Set aside time for choosing. When you do, you are saying, "This is my life. My health and self-esteem and how I age are all on the line."

Nothing changes until there is action. Planning promotes action. After planning we are free to act and are released from the dilemma of wondering what will happen next.

Without a plan, you fall prey to mind games. "That éclair looks good . . . irresistibly good. Maybe I shouldn't . . . Maybe I should. Lots of calories . . . I don't know." The internal debate is tiring and a trap. Having a plan cuts through it and you can tell yourself, "I don't have to think about this now. I'll just follow my plan. It's a good one and I have faith in it."

Coming up with your own plan is the best way to create your own experience and prevent things from "just happening" to throw you off course. Your course has been set by making intelligent, rational choices to move in the direction you've chosen. Planning is a tool for one of the most valuable forms of freedom you can experience via self-discipline.

PLAN TO PLAN!

Charlotte joined the Living Thin Program years ago when she was the Director of Admissions at the Johns Hopkins University School of Hygiene and Public Health. Charlotte not only fell in love with the program but she designed a brochure that is still used to highlight the responses of past students to the program. Charlotte wrote:

> I hated being heavy, but could not endure the boredom of dieting for very long. After trying many programs and following numerous diets, I found the one that treated me as an intelligent individual and consistently held my interest — Living Thin! I lost 55 pounds, have kept it off and gained new enthusiasm for work, relationships and living.

As Charlotte learned and began living the Rational Living component of the program, she elected to visit the REBT Institute in New York City. Her personal interpretation of Dr. Ellis's formula for rational thinking is presented in chart form on page 195.

ASSIGNMENT 4

Before you begin the assignment I want you to turn to Chapter 3 and read and reread the section on Motivation and Change.

Start by deciding which one of these habits relates to you and jot down, on a separate sheet of paper, your solution for each specific problem. Then examine Sylvia's solutions.

Habits List

1. When I start eating, I can't stop.

2. I taste everything-plus when I'm cooking.

3. Every time I pass through the kitchen, I grab something to eat.

4. I am usually eating or drinking while I am on the phone.

5. I enjoy eating while watching TV — which is quite often.

6. When I come home at the end of the day, I am usually ravenous and always overeat.

7. When I go to the movies, I usually indulge in popcorn or candy.

8. When I am driving, I eat if there is any food in the car.

9. Before I go to bed, I feel that I must have a snack.

10. When I am bored, angry, fatigued, depressed, or lonely I turn to food to make me feel better.

(ABOUT PARTIES)

11. When I am setting up a party and place the nuts and chips around, I tell myself I'll just take a few, but a few becomes a lot. When I see others snacking, I cannot resist doing the same, even if I don't want it. I usually overeat when I socialize.

12. I cannot pass up sweets whenever they are served.

13. When company leaves and I am cleaning up, I eat.

ABCs of Rational Emotive Therapy (also D and E)

A — Event

I went for a job interview and failed to get the job.

B — Headtalk (Irrational)

How awful to get rejected! I can't stand this rejection! This makes me a rotten person! I'll never get a good job. I'll always do badly on job interviews.

C — Feelings (Irrational)

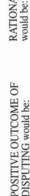

WORTHLESS! DEPRESSED! ANXIOUS! ANGRY! HOPELESS!

RATIONAL FEELINGS would be:
- Sorrow
- Regret
- Frustration
- Irritation
- Determination to keep trying

D — Disputing

Why is it awful to get rejected?
Why can't I stand this rejection?
How does this rejection make me a rotten person?
What is the evidence that I will never get a good job?
Why must I always do badly on job interviews?

POSITIVE OUTCOME OF DISPUTING would be:
- It is not awful — just inconvenient.
- I can stand it though I don't like it.
- Rejection does not make me a rotten person — but a person who needs improvement.
- It may be hard for me to find a good job — not impossible!
- I don't have to do badly on job interviews — if I learn from my mistakes and practice.

E — Choices

1. Refuse to go for other job interviews.
2. Continue to be depressed and anxious about getting a good job.
3. Abandon efforts to try.
4. Wail and whine.

RATIONAL CHOICES would be:
1. Continue to go on job interviews.
2. Look into upgrading my skills with additional training.
3. Send out more letters applying for jobs.
4. Register with an employment agency.
5. Role play the job interview.

 EVENT leads to

 FEELINGS because of intervening

 HEADTALK, or what I am saying to myself about

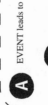

Solutions

1. *When I start I can't stop.*

    Planning is the key. Practice is what you need. However, do not expect perfection. Above all, refuse to feel guilty when you goof. All you need is awareness and willingness to practice. Read your notes about working around (not eliminating) your compulsive personality. You will make it if you refuse to give up.

2. *I taste everything-plus when I'm cooking.*

    As you prepare food in your kitchen, have several acceptable snacks on hand so you won't gorge on a pre-meal meal.

3. *Every time I pass through the kitchen, I grab something to eat.*

    Your average eating plan for the day includes breakfast, lunch, a snack between lunch and dinner, dinner and a snack before bedtime. You simply are not allowed to eat when you pass through the kitchen. It is just a terrible habit. Give it up or avoid the kitchen.

4. *I am usually eating or drinking while I am on the phone.*

    No eating while you are talking. It is rude and results in too many unnecessary calories. Give it up.

5. *I enjoy eating while watching TV which is quite often.*

    Eating while watching TV is okay in my book. I do it all the time. However, the secret lies in eating what you have planned to eat. Where you eat it is your business. I do not agree with authors who insist you eat in one place all the time. Too boring, too restrictive, doesn't work.

6. *When I come home at the end of the day, I am usually ravenous and always overeat.*

You're ravenous because you failed to have something in the middle of the day. The secret lies in not allowing yourself to be hungry. Thinking about this issue is what it takes. Remember you are vulnerable when you are hungry. Eating frequently is the key to your success.

7. *When I go to the movies, I usually indulge in popcorn or candy.*

Another rotten habit. You really can train yourself not to eat while you are watching a film. However, if you are entitled to a snack and choose to have it while you are at the movies, that's okay providing you can afford it. Avoid popcorn that is salted and buttered. If you insist, have it unbuttered and unsalted. Take it from me, if you go for the butter and salt, the damage will be painful. Incidentally, the same thing applies to saltines. The salt and the flour in a saltine causes an immediate water retention problem, which is terribly discouraging when you step on the scale. And stepping on a scale every day of your life is the healthiest thing you can do, providing you are educated enough to know what is happening.

8. *When I am driving I eat if there is any food in the car.*

Stop eating or drinking while driving. It is a great way to have an accident.

9. *Before I go to bed, I feel that I must have a snack.*

So have it. Just include it in your plan for the day. But remember to add some forceful self-talk: "That is all after the allotment."

10. *When I am bored, angry, fatigued, depressed or lonely, I turn to food to make me feel better.*

Eating when you are bored simply leaves you with two problems instead of one. Still bored but now also disgusted. Force yourself to resolve your boredom. You and you alone are responsible for your boredom. Make a list of enjoyable pursuits and do them. Refuse to feel sorry for yourself. Also, avoid eating when you are tired. Fatigue erodes your motivation. Rest or sleep, but don't eat when you are tired.

11. *When I am setting up a party and place the nuts and chips around, I tell myself I'll just take a few, but a few becomes a lot. When I see others snacking, I cannot resist doing the same even if I don't want it; I usually overeat when I socialize.*

Again, make a plan — with the understanding that goofing is okay. Reread the portion on bingeing and never stop enjoying your life.

12. *I cannot pass up sweets whenever they are served.*

Trust me when I tell you that anything goes — even whiskey — but not sweets. Avoid candy, cakes, ice cream LIKE THE PLAGUE. It will destroy whatever progress you make. It is a silent killer until you have reached your goal weight. Even then, though you may have it on occasion, know full well that sugar will always be an enemy that you can AT TIMES enjoy.

13. *When company leaves and I am cleaning up, I eat.*

If you cannot handle cleaning up without nibbling, use the garbage can. Load it all into the trash and be done with it. You are not a garbage can. That stuff is better off in the garbage can than in your stomach. Don't even consider donating it to the homeless; it will spoil before it ever reaches them.

Living Assertively Is An Art Form . . . Learn To Do It With Style

"No matter how upset I am, no matter how depressed, angry, anxious or guilt ridden, I have what it takes to change old eating habits if I am willing to make a firm commitment."

Right?

Well, yes, providing you know how to control and manage the DEGREE of your upsettedness. If you allow your negative emotions to overwhelm you, you will surely be unable to resist the goodies. At this point your desire to escape from your misery will probably be much stronger than your desire to lose weight. During these periods alcoholics turn to alcohol, druggies to drugs, smokers to cigarettes, and overeaters to food. What better than a slice of hot apple pie smothered in vanilla ice cream to reduce the pain of your depression or anger?

Be sure to turn to Chapter 2 if and when you need to refresh your Rational Thinking skills.

Regardless of how delicious or nutritious a food may be, changing a well-established eating pattern of any kind is a difficult task. Avoiding change is much easier. The more ammunition you have for making these changes, the simpler your task. A powerful tool for change of any kind is understanding and using the "Art" of Assertive Living. There is a dramatic connection between an assertive lifestyle and reaching your goal.

A part of my continuing fascination with my program stems from the information and knowledge I gain from the individuals with whom I work. They have told me *(and showed me)* how much they enjoyed the classes on assertion, aggression, and passivity and how they benefited from learning how closely connected these subjects are to changing eating and living habits.

Show me a bona fide, dyed-in-the-wool passive personality, and I will show you an individual who has more than an average number of problems in changing old habits. Clearly understanding the *importance* of distinguishing assertion from aggression and understanding the *connection* between passivity and approval seeking is vitally important to Living Thin. Its power will be evident on the scale when you weigh yourself.

Assertion — Why It Matters

Asserting yourself feels good. It feels good because when you assert yourself you are sharing *your* innermost feelings and thoughts with others.

Losing a relationship is one thing,
but losing yourself by abdicating your values
is the greatest loss of all.

Self-assertion simplifies life by clearing the air of the confusion and guesswork that comes from wishing others knew what you were thinking or knew what you wanted.

When you and I can communicate honestly and simply, it removes the uncertainty, the fog, the cloudiness that all too often stops people from understanding each other — or even worse — is responsible for the confusion and misunderstanding that damages relationships.

We live in a crazy mixed-up world that is full of uncertainty and confusion. I believe with all my heart that the saddest aspect of our world today is the way in which individuals are diminished by the pace of modern life and the technology that all but engulfs us. In a world that robs you of your individuality, where you are little more than a number, the way you feel, the measure of respect you have for yourself, becomes more important than ever. Developing the courage to speak up, to be heard has become even more important in developing self-confidence and self-esteem.

Kafka wrote his literary and philosophical tale "Metamorphosis" about the loss of individuality in the world as it becomes more and more modernized, technological, and dehumanized. He believed that when individuality is lost, you are lost.

If you fail to speak up, especially when an issue is important to you, you are sending a message to others that you don't think what you have to say matters, that you don't deserve to be heard, that what you want doesn't rate. What someone else thinks of you is more important than what you think of yourself.

It's important to know that a totally passive person is a rarity. By deciding to read this book, you are already telling me you are an assertive person. If you are being walked on, it is because you wait too long to do something about your frustrations, not because you can't do anything about them.

Granted, our world is full of tension, pressure, and anxiety, and having to learn the art of assertion is a task you'd rather not take on. However, if you are serious about change — in this instance losing weight healthily and forever — then let me assure you that acquiring assertive skills is one of the most powerful tools in your tool chest, one you cannot afford to be without.

For this reason, you need a clear understanding of what is meant when we talk about ASSERTION, PASSIVITY, and AGGRESSION, and how approval-seeking becomes a major player in this scenario.

Acting assertively means standing up for your rights and expressing what you believe, feel, and want in direct, honest, appropriate ways that respect the rights of others. What do we mean by "appropriate"? Simply, does it make sense to speak up at a particular time? For example, if your friend asks your opinion of a garment she's just had altered, and you think it makes her look like a hag, it would hardly be appropriate, or in good taste, to assert your opinion at this moment. In this instance you might choose to resort to a little restraint by agreeing it looked lovely.

When you insist on behaving passively, you make yourself a doormat for everyone around you. You feel "used" and worse. It leads to a loss of self-respect and very often to anger. That anger and disgust with yourself often leads to a hot fudge sundae. An overly passive personality is depressed more often than she would like to admit.

We know depression and passivity erode motivation for change. This fact and working on a solution requires a willingness to practice and work, work and practice, which is *essential* before you can even *think* about Living Thin and loving it.

The more passive I am the less motivated I am. Passive people take the path of least resistance — with themselves and with others. Some people may love your passivity simply because they are always getting what they want from you, but it doesn't mean that they respect you. REMEMBER, IN ALL RELATIONSHIPS WE ARE CONTINUALLY EDUCATING PEOPLE AROUND US ABOUT HOW WE WANT TO BE TREATED. THE RESPONSIBILITY IS YOURS, NOT THEIRS.

When Mary decides to avoid being assertive by choosing to behave passively, she is telling the world (and herself) that either she doesn't care enough about the issue or is fearful of expressing herself because of the consequences. Here is an example of how Mary's lack of assertion applies to her weight loss. Mary goes to a party knowing she can't handle a slice or even a taste of chocolate cake (she knows that skipping it is easier than just having a taste). Even though she has made a contract with herself not to eat the cake, she caves in when her friend and hostess insists she have a slice. Her inability to assert herself and follow through with her decision is evident both in her failure to forego the cake and her unwillingness to "stand up" to her hostess.

When Mary chooses to avoid expressing herself (to herself and others), she is telling herself — and the world — her attitudes about change; namely, change is not her top priority. By being passive she is choosing the "easy way"— the status quo — which leads to procrastination and erodes her motivation for change.

We are not suggesting that all passive people are overweight or that all passive people are unable to do hard things. All I am suggesting is that one way of feeling good about yourself is speaking up when an issue is important to you. And the better you feel about yourself, the more likely it will be easy to say "NO" to negative challenges such as a slice of chocolate cake.

Also, I am entirely aware that people are complex and that at times a passive person becomes aggressive or assertive or vice versa. My point is simply this: THE BETTER YOU FEEL ABOUT YOURSELF, THE EASIER YOUR TASK.

By waiting too long to express your feelings about important issues, you wind up feeling helpless and at times exploited. At this point it's natural for your anger to escalate and you just may wind up making unhealthy decisions that could have been avoided had you spoken up earlier. One day while working on this book, my office manager began reacting passively to a situation that erupted in the office. Each day she found that she had little opportunity to complete a given task before being assigned four other tasks. Instead of asserting herself, she began feeling angry and, at one point, without any explanation, allowed her anger to overtake her. She threw her keys down and walked out without further ado.

Since I pride myself on practicing what I preach, I insisted we discuss what was bothering her and exhorted her to assert herself and share her feelings with me, since I was entirely unaware of them. She did and we resolved the dilemma easily and quickly.

How does "aggression" differ from "assertion"? Aggression involves reaching a goal with no regard or respect for others. Humiliating or attacking someone is acceptable and serves to intimidate on the way to reaching that goal. In other words, *anything goes as long as it serves my purpose.* While aggression is preferable to passivity, it *guarantees* alienating others.

> No set of rules works for everyone. Knowing what you want is 50 percent of the battle.

The major issue here is remembering the differences between assertion and aggression. Often the difference lies only in
style. In other words, the assertive person considers reaching a
goal but always with tact, sensitivity, and a high regard for the
feelings of others. For instance, if your goal is to fire an employee who has failed to perform up to standards, you would in-
form the employee, with sensitivity, the reasons for his dis-
missal so he could perhaps benefit from the experience. This
beats announcing, "You're Fired!" and storming out the door.

Respect for others and care for their feelings is the missing
element in aggression.

At times the difference between assertion and aggression
lies only in the tone of voice. The same remark, spoken softly,
loses its aggressive quality. The quality of your relationships
will rise and fall on your skill in this area.

Being assertive is the ideal stance because you're being honest with yourself and others and increasing your chances of getting what you want. Aggression is not as desirable as assertion
because you're continually alienating others and thus decreasing
your chances for getting what you want. Passivity is the lowest
of the three, unless an individual is passive by choice, which is
entirely different than being passive by default. Why you're
being passive is the key. If a person is passive by choice, that is
perfectly healthy. If a person is passive for fear of hurting or
alienating others, that is unhealthy because this individual is
going to walk away frustrated — decreasing the chances of getting what he wants. In other words these people are cowardly.

Here are a couple of questions to ask yourself about the
value of asserting yourself in your relationships:

1. How will our relationship work on a long-term basis if I fail
    to say what I want or believe?

2. Will the long-term results be worse than the short-term discomfort I may feel by being assertive?

When you assert yourself, you are simply exercising your rights to say, "This is who I am. This is how I feel. This is what I believe. And we both have the privilege to enjoy these rights in a healthy relationship."

Sounds good, doesn't it? It is and it works!

Change Isn't Easy, But Not Changing is Harder

Passive people usually have much difficulty losing weight. Why? Passive people are continually giving themselves negative messages that interfere with change. For example, *"I've tried before and I know it won't work."* But changing a lifestyle takes a lot of doing, energy, time, belief, and confidence — elements often lacking in passive personalities. Change requires awareness, commitment, a lot of practice, and ABOVE ALL — A HIGH LEVEL OF MOTIVATION. Motivation and passivity are mutually exclusive and completely incompatible.

We know that it takes strong desire and motivation to behave differently. Why is this the case? Because remaining "as is" is so much more comfortable. But there may be other aspects of your personality that are serious obstacles to making change. We will explore them now.

Obstacle #1 : Fear of Displeasing Others

The key to overcoming this hurdle is understanding that regardless of how kind, passive, generous, talented, or handsome you may be, you will never please everyone all the time.

In my class, I used to introduce this portion by saying, "I know it's hard to believe, but even I can't 'make it' with everyone." It always got a good laugh. Believe me, even the most charismatic people, from Lana Turner to Ted Turner, fail at times to please everyone.

Wanting approval is natural. We all want others to like us and approve of us because it feels good to know that we are liked. We all enjoy praise and compliments, and it is reassuring to be stroked. It is only when we find ourselves *needing* approval rather than *wanting* approval that we are in trouble. An excessive need for approval usually results in having to give up a part of ourselves.

When you become that needy, you might as well be wearing a badge that invites people to abuse you. You wind up feeling good about yourself only when "they" approve of you. If and when that need for approval extends to not only one individual but to everyone with whom you come in contact, you are in big trouble. That need must GO if you want to make changes in your way of life.

One of the favorite stories I used in my classes was the story of "Phyllis." Phyllis is your best friend. She has a physical disability that causes her to sway awkwardly when she walks. You love her and she has become an important part of your life. She surprises you one day by saying, "It would make me feel better if you would agree to drop your left shoulder when we go out together because it would make my infirmity look less serious."

While you are not happy about walking around with a dropped shoulder, you tell yourself, "Big deal, I'll drop it if it makes her feel so much better. Why not?" Well, it doesn't take very long for Phyllis to ask you to drop your shoulder just a few inches more. Before you know it you are walking around with your shoulder way down. And you know what? Phyllis disappears because she found a friend who is a better bridge player than you are, and now you've developed a habit of stooping over to the side. So beware how low you are willing to stoop to keep anyone, even your best friend.

Before you can move on to becoming more assertive you first want to cope with your need for approval. Why? Because it leads to a dead end. There is no way you will give yourself permission to become more assertive if you are being victimized by your need for approval or your fear of being rejected.

There is virtually no way you can move through life without having others disapprove of you at times. Even at critical times. If you decide to give your right eye to a deserving child so she can have vision, there will be some people who will disapprove of your decision.

If you find yourself turning to others often, ask yourself if you are saying that their opinion is more important to you than your own. Too many people feel depressed, anxious, and upset when significant people fail to approve of what they do or say. If, in your relationships, you are labeled "uncaring" or "selfish" because you choose to behave in a certain way, that relationship is designed to make you feel guilty for any form of independence you may show.

> Whoever has the responsibility holds the power.

But that very independence about important (and lesser) matters is the basis of being in charge of your life, i.e., being assertive, honest, and faithful to yourself! Unfortunately, we live in a society that discourages people from thinking for themselves. Consider television commercials: you are urged to purchase mouthwash, panty hose, exercise equipment, clothing, and cars that have famous names on them. Advertisers understand that most people feel more secure when a product is endorsed by a company or a famous person — as though that guarantees quality. How is the issue of food connected to this problem? What about the issue of low-cal or low fat foods?

In a previous chapter I talked about how these items can often make you fat and sick. Learn to THINK for yourself. The companies that sell these items are interested in sales. Your interest lies in your health. It doesn't make sense to lose weight if the price is poor health. Eating low-cal foods surely won't guarantee weight loss. (I know, I tried eating low-cal foods for years without success. The fewer the calories, the more I ate.)

It's also important to remember that an item marked "low fat" doesn't mean the item is healthy. The manufacturer may have substituted a chemical to replace the taste of fat. THINK before you make your purchase. Are you sure you will be healthier and thinner by choosing low fat, low-cal foods, or are you merely buying psychological messages that often fail to work? Be assertive about food choices, about foods you are choosing to feed to your family and friends. Use healthy, slender people as role models. Watch them. You will learn much. Above all, think and be assertive when making your food choices. You may be happier eating less of the good stuff. The choice is always yours.

"I've been passive for such a long time. Switching gears means making changes, and change means work, energy . . . WOW! However, if I do decide to make these changes, where do I start? Where do I begin?"

First, just jot down the pluses of living more assertively. Think hard about situations in which you have often wished you had been more assertive. Once you identify them and situations like them, you can actively work on being more assertive with your friends, family, and co-workers. You can express your desires in a honest, open manner. Here are a few examples:

a. Telling your hostess how much you love her but that you cannot afford to even taste her delicious "to die for" desserts.

b. Making assertive food decisions when planning a party. Choose healthy foods that are also tasty. Educate your friends. YOU make the choices. Refuse to be influenced ONLY by their wishes. Select foods that reflect your interest in health and weight loss, or have a choice of both.

c. Developing the habit of "speaking up" and asking for what you want — meeting places, restaurants, airports, foreign countries, etc. Plan ahead and "speak up." You'll be both pleased and happier with your choices.

d. Expressing your feelings to your mother about your relationship so that her expectations for you are more reasonable.

e. Returning a garment you have no intention of wearing. So you made a mistake, SO WHAT!

I recall attending a seminar at the REBT Institute in New York some years ago led by Dr. Ellis. I remember vividly one exercise he suggested for getting passive personalities to begin asserting themselves. Get on a subway and yell, "Broadway and 42nd Street" loudly and with authority. You will discover that many people will simply ignore you, while a few may dismiss you as being slightly wacky. But the lesson is invaluable. We worry so much about what others think of us instead of realizing that most people aren't thinking about us at all. They are naturally more concerned about themselves than they are about you. This type of lesson helps to free you from being unduly concerned about the whole issue of approval from others.

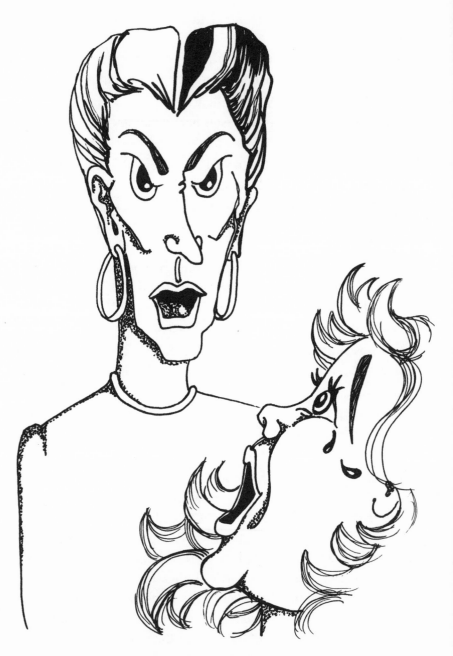

I don't like you.

Change involves cultivating effective habits. Choose the behavior you want to change. Make a plan about when and where. Make a mental plan. See yourself going to the movies and refusing to eat while you view the film regardless of what your friend is doing. Practice and remember that going back to square one doesn't mean you've failed. Simply trust the process and refuse to give up.

No matter who you are or what type of lifestyle you choose, there is no way you can escape some disapproval. By expecting it, it becomes less of a problem. Here are some examples of approval-seeking behavior:

- Backing down from your beliefs because someone else disapproves
- "Sucking up" to others
- Calling someone else "selfish" because you are jealous
- Gossiping for attention
- Clamming up because you suspect someone else will contradict you
- Nonconforming for the sake of remaining "in"

> The only approval you need is your own!

Why do we insist on hanging on to our need for approval? How can we make "change" possible?

The Living Thin Program is based on a process of identifying our feelings, examining the connection between the thoughts in our heads (our self-talk) and the irrational and self-defeating behaviors they produce, and then challenging and, hopefully, eradicating the negative head talk. It requires practice and determination to then replace those thoughts with a rational thinking pattern that will help move you into healthy behaviors.

Here is an example that relates to approval seeking.

A. Situation — Miriam and I are working together on a very public project that depends on the support of people who see us as a unit. From the start we had several differences of opinions, but as work progressed the differences grew. She then decided she no longer cares for me and has walked away from the project.

B. Your Thoughts — *"This is terrible. I should have agreed with her more often. What will others say about the breakup? She should have stuck it out. I can't stand the thought of what others will say about the breakup."*

C. Your Feelings — Depressed, anxious, guilty. It is important to remember that it is not A, the situation, that causes the depression, anxiety, and guilt. It is B, the head talk that causes it.

D. Identify, then vigorously challenge, question, and examine your head talk. The process might be something like this: *"It is disappointing but hardly terrible. It would be lovely if I had responded to her criticism, but since I am a fallible human being, and even if I had responded perfectly, I would have probably goofed elsewhere at another time. It's probably just as well that it happened now. While I would enjoy having the approval of everyone, I can make do with whatever approval I pick up on the way as long as I have my own."*

Then there are choices to make.

Choice 1. I can assertively confront my friend about the issue and attempt to repair the situation.

Choice 2. I can choose to accept the situation passively and let it go, understanding that choosing to be passive is as valid as choosing to be assertive.

Choice 3. I can choose to neither confront nor accept the situation but rather to "wail and whine."

The issue is I AM RESPONSIBLE FOR MY FEELINGS, NOT MIRIAM. If Miriam is responsible for my being upset, then I will need Miriam to be responsible if I want to change how I feel. YOU CAN TAKE CONTROL OF YOUR UPSETTEDNESS. WHEN YOU BLAME OTHERS FOR YOUR FEELINGS, YOU GIVE THEM CONTROL. If your feelings are controlled by what others say, think, and do then you become helpless, victimized by their behavior.

Hanging onto irrational thinking patterns makes it easier to avoid change. Avoiding the responsibility for change is at the core of unhealthy thinking and behaving. If you give up blaming others and needing others so much, you have no choice than to risk growing up and taking control of your life. ARE YOU READY TO GROW UP?

Here are some self-defeating thoughts/thinking patterns that will chain you to the past and allow you to avoid change:

- *"That is just the way I am. I've always been like this"*
- *"It's just my nature to be so sensitive to how other people feel"*
- *"I can't help it. I can't change"*

If you insist on repeating these statements, I promise you they will stop you from growing and changing and lock you into a lifestyle that is not to your liking.

However, if you challenge and question your head talk, you will find yourself feeling distressed less often. Your goal is not becoming an unemotional person, but rather to learn how to control overreacting so you can think and behave rationally.

Obstacle #2: Fear of Rejection in Social Situations

*"Suppose I ask her or him for a date and the answer is 'no.'
Wouldn't that be awful?"*

Disappointing, but hardly awful. This example of WHAT-IF-ITIS demonstrates the lack of logic of those who fear rejection. The fear of being rejected results in losing out on what might be, in some instances, interesting or important relationships.

My favorite story about rejection took place many years ago during a visit to the La Costa Spa. During my stay, I decided to talk to the hostess to tell her that while I was content during the day while I was busy with golf, I did not enjoy eating alone at dinner, especially when the lights in the dining room were so dim that I couldn't even read.

As we spoke, a woman approached to whom I said, "I saw you eating alone last night. Would you like to join me for dinner this evening?" To which she replied, "No, I would not." To which I replied, "You don't know what you're missing." The hostess was embarrassed and turned and invited me to meet her in the lounge later. When we met, she apologized for the woman's behavior and said, "I know how badly you must have felt." I replied, "I didn't feel rejected. She doesn't even know me, so how could she reject me?"

The hostess said, "You are so right. She happens to be a buyer at Saks Fifth Avenue, and she is inundated with women. She comes here four times a year to get away from them."

Remember Eleanor Roosevelt's comment: "No one can upset you or reject you without your permission." If you absorb this one lesson and practice the skills to overcome this obstacle, you will be way ahead of the game.

Obstacle #3: Fear of Hurting Others' Feelings

In this case, you are assuming that the person you are talking to cannot handle an honest, up-front conversation. Then you tell yourself that you are too caring to tell the other person the truth.

When you do so, you are potentially insulting this person by your assumption. Admit it: it's not their feelings you're trying to spare. More truthfully you are justifying your passive nature because it is easier than changing it. That means YOU GET WHAT YOU ACCEPT, and for passive people that means no risk — NO CHANGE.

> The fact that old habits die hard doesn't mean they shouldn't die.

The common denominator of all these obstacles — the fear of displeasing others, the fear of being rejected, and the fear of hurting someone's feelings — is that they all cement you to your passive behaviors. What I am challenging you to see is that you may be hiding behind these fears to justify avoiding (and changing) your passivity!

The passive person's reasoning is based on the underestimation of his or her own value, in other words, low self-worth. The cycle is clear. Passivity based on low self-regard leads to feeling sorry for yourself, which can lead directly to the cookie jar. Being passive locks you into this loser's game where you accept (even anticipate) your losses with the understanding that you don't have the right (or the right stuff) to behave assertively.

This vicious, self-defeating cycle maintains the status quo: by risking nothing, you gain nothing. In baseball terms: no runs, no hits, no errors. It also invites the other team to come up to bat and take their best shot at winning.

The lesson here is to avoid the excesses of both passive and aggressive behaviors. The beauty of assertive behavior is that it avoids the pitfalls of both passivity and aggression while maximizing opportunities to honestly express yourself. I simply cannot tell you how grateful I am for the training in these areas I received that helped me overcome obstacles in so many areas of my life.

If your failure to control your weight is connected to your attitudes, here is your Basic Assertive Bill of Rights:

1. The right to act in ways that promote my health, dignity, and self-respect — and to grant this right to others.
2. The right to be treated with respect.
3. The right to say "no" without feeling guilty.
4. The right to change my mind.
5. The right to ask for what I want.
6. The right to do less than I am capable of doing.
7. The right to make mistakes.
8. The right to think I am terrific.

Old Habits Die Hard

While many class participants became quite enthusiastic about the newfound assertion, they found soon enough that old habits do indeed die hard and that change cannot happen immediately. Patience, awareness, and a desire to work at change is what change is about. Avoid having unreasonable expectations. Start slowly and gradually. Be willing to experiment. Have fun with it. Be daring. Be bold. The thrill of moving forward brings so much reward that the work and practice will seem insignificant. You'll never achieve "perfection," so relax and enjoy the journey. And accept the indisputable fact that regardless of how assertive you become, you will never, and I mean never, control the universe. You will never have the power to make Tuesday follow Sunday. Absolutely no way can you control your friends or your children (especially your children). Try, as the famous saying goes, to be willing to work at changing those things we don't like, to accept the things we cannot change, and somehow find the wisdom to know the difference.

We're back to freeing ourselves from our "shoulds," "musts," and "oughts" when we choose to be assertive with ourselves and accept the fact that we upset ourselves with the demands we make on ourselves and others. When you've practiced and managed to internalize these very basic concepts, you will be on your way to becoming your own therapist.

Assertive Attitudes

To become an assertive individual, you need first to know yourself. Why? Because the issue of assertion is a personal experience. The more you know about yourself the more adept you become at identifying the ways in which assertion can be of value to you. Though it is not the answer or solution for each and every problem, it is an important tool that you simply cannot do without.

The goal of "knowing yourself" is to accept who you are in order to work with your limitations, preferences, and strengths rather than to unrealistically force yourself against the grain.

How To Determine the Categories Into Which You Fit

By becoming aware of your body language (which may account for 80 percent of how and what you communicate), how you come across to others (the messages you are sending), your expectations, your reactions, and the reactions others have to you, you will have a clearer grasp of "who you are."

Carefully review the following chart and see if you can recognize which style has your name on it. Practice saying, "I don't agree with you" in the same tone and with the same body language described below, and you will see how many different ways there are to say the same thing.

BODY LANGUAGE/TONE	MESSAGE
Aggressive. Contemptuous tone.	I not only don't agree with you, I think you're not too bright. I am not going to change my opinion.
Assertive. Controlled and even tone of voice. Good eye contact.	I mean what I say. I do not agree with you but that we disagree does not bother me.
Passive. Ingratiating tone. Very soft. On the apologetic side. Eyes averted. Speaks· with a lot of hesitation.	If I disagree, it is done almost apologetically. I am fearful of making you angry or upsetting you.

The assertive person is generally self-assured and is mildly emphatic about his/her views. The aggressive person usually conveys an air of self-importance and superiority and is overbearing. The passive person clearly lacks self-confidence and appears anxious. Their messages come through in fuzzy or contradictory ways. For example, they may laugh while saying, "I am really angry at you."

Now, let's compare passive, assertive, and aggressive personalities in terms of behaviors that are typical of each and in terms of the emotional content, response, outcomes and payoffs that these behaviors elicit.

Two questions you may be asking yourself: How can you tell when you have become more assertive? What can you do to not allow yourself to become discouraged?

ANSWER: If in the past you *always* responded passively and now you find yourself responding assertively on occasion. THAT IS IMPROVEMENT!

ANSWER: Accept yourself assertively. Encourage yourself assertively. Be brave. Be willing to experiment. Practice saying "NO" even when you may want to say yes. Ask yourself how it feels. Be patient. And above all — ENJOY THE CHANGE.

Self-Interest is Not Selfishness

Rabbi Hillel asked long ago, "If I am not for me, who will be? And if I am not for others, what good am I?" This query captures the essence of a difficult dilemma. Let's examine this issue for a moment.

Many people define an individual who pursues a healthy lifestyle as selfish. What they mean is the person is too concerned with himself, too self-absorbed with the way he eats, thinks, and looks. He has a what's-in-it-for-me attitude.

Ann has a bright, articulate, attractive, vibrant personality. She is very much concerned with her physical and emotional health. She is interested in and absorbed in healthy eating habits. She spends time at the health food stores. She reads about organic foods. She knows about junk foods. She engages in some form of exercise daily and is vitally absorbed in a variety of interests. She attends classes and teaches. DOES THIS PRECLUDE ANN FROM BEING A GOOD MOTHER? Is she as interested in her children's activities and interests as her own?

	Passive	Assertive	Aggressive
Behavior Trait	Reluctant to express wants, ideas and feelings. Expresses them in self-deprecating ways.	Espresses wants, ideas and feelings in direct and appropriate ways.	Same as assertive but at the expense of others.
Goal	To please	To communicate	To dominate and humiliate
Your Feelings: Why You Act This Way	Disappointed with self. Often angry and resentful. May feel like comforting yourself with hot-fudge sundae.	Confident. Feel good about yourself.	Self-righteous, superior. Sometimes regretful later.
Others' Feelings About Themselves When You Act This Way	Guilty or superior	Respected, valued	Humiliated, hurt
Others' Feelings About You When You Act This Way	Irritation, pity, disgust	Usually respected	Angry, vengeful
Outcome of Behavior	Don't get what you want. Anger builds. You eat more and more and exercise less and less. Gain weight easily.	Often get what you want.	Often get what you want but all too often you alienate others.
Payoff of Behavior	Avoids confrontations, immediate conflict and tension.	Feel good about yourself. Increased self-respect, confidence, and respect of others. Healthier relationships. More determined to reach goal weight. Steadies and boosts motivation.	Gets rid of your anger. Feel superior. Fully confident you can reach goal weight.

Does this mean she is not equally concerned with her husband and is not a spectacular bed partner? Of course not.

Hillary, on the other hand, thinks, speaks, and is absorbed only in her family. She is overweight. Not concerned with her appearance, she is a bit of a slob — indifferent to her looks. Her interests are centered only about her family — her husband's and children's interests. You can imagine how she feels about the Anns of this world.

Does this mean Hillary is unbalanced? Surely a balance is possible. Neither Ann nor Hillary need to be the models. Unless you are moderately healthy physically and emotionally, you can't be of any value to others. Back to moderation and common sense. A degree of selfishness is healthy and an excess is not.

Let's not forget the individual who enjoys giving so much to others that when she does not receive the applause and appreciation she demands (her head talk), she becomes neurotic. It is vital to accept that what we give to others is a choice — nothing more, nothing less. Since the giving is a choice, we need to be reasonable about our expectations.

Behaviorists tell us that relationships are apt to deteriorate rather than improve when people make excessive sacrifices to please another person. Understanding clearly the shadings and differences between selfishness and self-interest is very important. Passive individuals often use excuses to rationalize their deeply rooted desire to AVOID asserting themselves both verbally or physically. If you don't understand the difference between self-interest and selfishness, you will feel guilty whenever someone (especially someone close to you) asks you for a favor and

> **Never let "Hard to Do" get in the way of something worth doing.**

you refuse. Or, you will feel put out when you find yourself doing more than you really care to do.

Let's relate the issues of self-interest and selfishness to problems that arise as we endeavor to change our eating habits. Elizabeth, your dearest friend, gives a dinner party. Even though she knows how eager you are to succeed at losing weight and how vulnerable you are around sweets, she nevertheless insists that you try a slice of her chocolate pie, which she has prepared for the party. Elizabeth is concerned with Elizabeth, and while she has a right to behave in this manner, you, as a passive personality, may find it easier to "give in" to her request for a variety of reasons. First, "giving in" is easier than asserting yourself with Elizabeth. Two, Elizabeth and others may think you are "selfish" for going it alone, for not going along with the rest. If you truly know in your heart of hearts that you cannot handle "tastes," is it really selfish to speak up and say, *"How delicious that pie looks. If only I were not working so hard to get rid of my sweet tooth . . . I KNOW, I can't handle a taste . . . I'd want the whole pie. But the time will come when I will be begging for a piece of your delicious pie. I simply need to wait until I can afford that luxury."* Do you really think you would be acting selfishly? The issue of self-interest is closely related to self-respect.

If you don't like the word "self-interest," call it whatever you prefer. Intelligent and caring assertiveness means having respect for, and valuing yourself. To be specific it means:

1. Limiting what you are willing to do for others.

2. Understanding what is appropriate and what is not appropriate.

3. Being reasonable about expectations of both self and others.

4. Refusing to become excessively upset with others or yourself.

5. Enjoying small changes and refusing to become greedy about what you choose to change.

6. Absolutely refusing to feel miserable when someone treats you unfairly.

7. Understanding clearly the consequences of being overwhelmed by incidents or circumstances.

8. Overlooking your imperfections as well as those of others.

What I am advocating is taking an assertive attitude toward your health by making assertive decisions and choices about daily health care, food, portion control, exercise, and your emotional health. All these issues play a major role in designing a healthy lifestyle.

Why is losing weight and keeping it off so difficult? We know how easy it is to turn to food when we are not feeling too good about ourselves. This is why being assertive is a vital tool in making healthy lifestyle changes. By that I mean assertive choices about food, exercise, and communication that are based on a healthy respect for yourself.

It is not a black and white issue. At times we are all passive, aggressive, and assertive. But clearly understanding the differences and learning to be in charge of your reactions, give you the ammunition to handle your interactions and your relationship with yourself.

Learning to Assert Yourself

If you tolerate treatment you feel you don't deserve for too long, you will grow bitter and resentful before you stand up for your rights. The issue is not whether, but WHEN! Healthy people don't wait forever before asserting themselves. A healthy person is properly concerned about his or her welfare and says, "I am perfectly capable of asserting myself now, so why wait for years to do it?"

Every passive person is capable of asserting himself whenever he chooses to do so. Saying that you failed to assert yourself because "it is not in my nature," is untrue. If someone were planning to burn down your home, would you stand by and do nothing, call no one because you were afraid of asserting yourself? Definitely not! If your child were being bullied by a person twice his size, would you not assert yourself even though you might get hurt? You would take action of some kind because you would be saying to yourself, "I cannot stand by. I will not allow this to happen."

> Our life is what our thoughts make it.
>
> Marcus Aurelius

In other words, no one is passive ALL THE TIME. It is merely a matter of how much pressure is brought to bear to motivate you. The lesson is you need not wait until so much pressure exists that you are desperate. When you know what you want, use your desire to do something about it.

Asking, "Why do passive people wait?" is a good question. Paul Hauck, an expert on the subject and one of the best teachers of REBT, has said that "passive people think they are forced to be passive. They believe they must accept being dominated by others, that they have no choice, and they have nothing to say about the matter.

To buttress Hauck's contention, consider the following: If someone is holding a gun to your head, then you really have no choice but to be passive when you are told, "You will be my psychological slave," because you could get your head blown off. But passive people often let others walk on them and take

> ## When you're through changing, you're through.
>
> Bruce Barton

advantage of them shamelessly because they are afraid. Afraid of what, you may well ask?

"Suppose I speak up and make a fool of myself."
"Suppose I speak up and no one listens."
"Suppose I speak up and someone laughs."

Okay, suppose someone laughs. So what? Can you stand it? What if your feelings are strong and your fears cause you to remain passive? How do you feel now? There is no guarantee that no one will laugh or not listen. They may or may not. The only guarantee is that if you don't speak up over issues that are important to you, eventually you lose your self-respect.

CHOICES are what we are urging you to think about. Not all situations warrant your speaking up. If I am on my way to a meeting and the traffic is heavy and moving slowly, why speak up, even if I have an opportunity to tell my friend (who is in the car) how I feel. Because it's just too unimportant. Save strong feelings for important issues. Why speak up when an elderly lady steps in front of you at the grocery store? Perhaps she didn't really see you and even if she did, so what?

There are times when "speaking up" is of exquisite importance, just as there are times when speaking up is stupid, when the consequences or outcomes simply don't deserve the effort. You make the call. What issues are important to you? After all, you are the central character in this skit. How do YOU feel about each issue? Only you can determine the behavior that causes you to feel as you do. You're with yourself all the time. Make the choices that work for you. But remember, YOU DO HAVE CHOICES. YOU ARE NOT "AVOIDING" UNLESS YOU CHOOSE TO.

Relationships — Expect Trouble Ahead

When you do decide to speak up, to be more assertive, be prepared for a bit of a rough ride when it comes to personal relationships — especially with people who are not accustomed to your being assertive. When you stand up to your boss, mate, or friends they will be surprised AND NATURALLY WON'T LIKE IT! They probably have been getting their way with you for a long time and will rebel against your assertive skills.

Be ready to fight for your rights. If you can hold on, stick to your guns, negotiate, and avoid aggression. The situation will improve, and people will respect you and begin treating you as an equal. Only rarely will you find someone who is mature enough to understand and accept the new you immediately.

As you begin changing, you will make mistakes. It is a natural tendency to feel guilty, but refuse to do so. Give yourself time. Accept that you are a beginner with these new skills in this exciting new world you are creating for yourself and don't expect yourself to be perfect. It will be helpful for you to be mindful of the rights of others as you assert your own rights.

Here are three ways of declining a dinner invitation when you have existing plans. Which way do you think is preferable?

Passive Pearl finds it easier to say "yes" than "no." She then feels guilty because she agreed to go, angry at herself for failing to say "no," and resentful of her date, too.

Aggressive Agnes receives the same invitation and responds, "You have a lot of nerve asking me to come to your home when

I've told you repeatedly why I need to stay home. You have no consideration and are the most selfish person I've met. Of course I am not coming. Forget it!"

Assertive Andrea says, "I would like to come to your home for dinner and hope you will invite me again, but it is impossible for me to make it this evening."

Andrea's response is healthy for these reasons: She is clear about where her priorities lie, she is unafraid of expressing her desire to refuse the invitation, and she declines with style. Refusal also says, while I *prefer* to have your approval, I don't *need* it.

Developing an Awareness of What Needs Changing

Arriving at this part of my Living Thin saga takes me back to the very beginning of my Living Thin days. I recall approaching my mentor, Dr. Hauserman-Campbell, about the possibility of my redesigning the program and teaching it myself. She assured me it would never work, that I was much too aggressive and abrasive to deal with people who were overweight. She assured me that overweight men and women, especially the women, could not work with an aggressive personality.

Dr. Hauserman-Campbell told me I'd have to change my personality. And guess what? With her help, I did! Not only did it make a big difference in the work I began doing, but it also helped me in many other areas of my life as well. At the time in question I was totally unaware of having a problem. I had to be told. How can somebody fix a problem if they are not even aware of having one? If you have a hole in your stocking and can't see it yourself, you will walk around with that hole that everyone can see but you. Think about the many people you know who have personality problems that cause them untold anguish and aren't even aware of their problems. The word is AWARENESS!

Accept the fact that nearly all people have a talent for behaving passively, assertively, or aggressively. Very often the behavior we choose depends on the situation. For my purposes, I am concentrating on helping you clearly understand the differences and shadings so that you will be able to switch from passive choices to more assertive ones in your quest for a healthier lifestyle. Suffice it to say that assertion and change will always be more compatible than passivity and change. THE VERY NATURE OF PASSIVITY SQUELCHES YOUR DESIRE AND MOTIVATION TO CHANGE.

What Does it Take to Become More Assertive?
The Living Thin Blueprint

Do you want to become more assertive? Do you wish, secretly or openly, that you could behave more assertively at times? If the answer is "yes," a good place to start is forcing yourself to "speak up" on occasion — even planning for it. Suppose you asked your waiter to toast your bagel dark but he brings it back toasted light. Make yourself look him in the eye and assertively ask him to bring it back toasted dark. Begin with small assignments, and like any other change or challenge, as you make yourself do it, you gain confidence, and the next time is not quite as difficult. It won't be long before you are telling your spouse that if he or she wants high calorie, unhealthy foods, he or she will have to order them when you dine out; he won't get them at home. And don't expect him to like the change. But if you are strong, refuse to give up, you will feel wonderful about yourself. Soon you will win the respect of others as you become more willing to "speak up" on matters that are truly important to you. When you question the wisdom of making these "changes," think of the consequences — the feelings of increased confidence and the respect you will win, and you will find the choices easier to make.

Assertiveness is based on:

- A willingness to value yourself as well as others
- A willingness to accept that at times you will NOT get your way
- A willingness to accept that there is no perfection, i.e., there is no perfect response for each and every situation
- A willingness to avoid expecting magic or pat answers for complex situations
- A willingness to settle for small, reasonable goals

Wanting APPROVAL from others is as natural as breathing, but always remember that WINNING your own APPROVAL comes first. Don't expect others to think well of you if you don't think well of yourself. At the same time keep two issues in mind:

1. It's unreasonable to expect close friends and family to accept your "new" person. Change is also difficult for them, and they have the freedom, the right, to dislike the new you. Be willing to hang in. They will change, and those who refuse to accept the new "you," well, they were never there for you to begin with.

2. Change takes time. Force yourself to be patient.

Esteem, Assertiveness, and Confidence

In my Living Thin classes, I'd often pose the question, "If I only had one gift to give my children, what would it be?" A big hunk of self-acceptance (assuming they had their health). The ability to love and accept themselves for who they are — warts, idiosyncrasies, extra pounds, and all. Where can you get this good stuff? Is it for sale at Neiman Marcus or Saks Fifth Avenue? No it is not. It's a rare commodity.

The next gift would have to be self-esteem. Call it self-confidence, self-efficacy — a belief in your abilities.

Here is a simple formula for self-esteem: Every day do something hard, something boring, something for someone else (without mentioning it), and something for yourself. Studies have proved conclusively that individuals can work and practice to overcome nearly any habit they wish to change including the habit of passivity. BUT CHANGE FIRST REQUIRES A STRONG AWARENESS OF THE NEED FOR CHANGE COUPLED WITH A STRONG DESIRE TO ACHIEVE THAT CHANGE. What then does it take for a person to be motivated enough to do whatever needs to be done to achieve change?

Let's begin with the issue of self-esteem. Everyone admires and respects an individual who clearly has a good opinion of himself. I'll never forget Dr. Fisher, president of Towson University in Baltimore, discussing a colleague, Dr. Buzz Shaw, now chancellor of Syracuse University. "Buzz really has it together," he said. "When he walks into a room you just know he knows who he is, where he is going, and that he will get there." I have often thought about Dr. Shaw and others who clearly had that quality; they knew what they wanted and they were willing to do the things they had to do to arrive at their destination.

What would it take for you to feel great about yourself? Have you accepted the message, "I can if I choose to?" What a great feeling, a wondrous gift, when you truly believe that! What would happen for you to feel really "good" about yourself? Make a list outlining the problems and the proposed solutions. For example, for me to feel good about me I would have to:

Problem	*Solution*
1. Lose weight	Put that eating chart on your fridge and respect it. Honor it.
2. Find a new beau	Work on it and if you can't find Harry, take John. Be willing to compromise.
3. Find a new friend	Join four new groups. Force yourself.
4. Get more exercise	Begin with a five minute walk, every day. Be reasonable with the amount, but do something every day.

Self-confidence is something you earn. As I wrote this book, there were times that I pretended to be more confident than I really felt. Let me tell you, it never hurt. In fact, the pretense often helped me to feel more confident. The response you elicit from a listener is influenced by your belief in what you are saying. If you are not confident in what you are saying, don't expect your listener to have confidence in you.

For the added edge in feeling good about ourselves, speaking with confidence and expressing yourself easily are important tools that will serve you well. The basis of confidence is realizing, and telling yourself, that no matter what the outcome you will continue to approve of your efforts, continue to work at it, and love yourself for who you are — unconditionally.

When you have that foundation, plus an understanding of when and where you are at your best, you will quite naturally see yourself in a positive light. That is when others will see you shine too.

Marie, for example, knows she is far from perfect. But she has a wonderful sense of herself. She accepts herself and enjoys herself. She knows she is a wonderful hostess and feels terrific about herself when she is entertaining others. This is quite different from neurotic approval seeking. Marie is showing off because she is already in her element, not because she desires the recognition from being in the spotlight.

As I think about the times I feel most confident, I realize that the same situations could apply to my readers. Each of us needs to discover the special areas in which our confidence is strongest by taking an inventory of our past experiences and using our intuition. My list is as follows:

1. Being with people I know or who know something about me before I meet them.

2. Teaching others. To me this means that I am prepared and anticipate an enjoyable experience — I can make a difference.

3. When the needle on the scale is where I want it to be.

4. When I am feeling physically fit. This comes from knowing that I am keeping up with the basic requirements for good physical health.

5. When I am feeling emotionally fit. This comes from knowing that I am in charge of the thinking that produces my feelings and behaviors.

When and where do I find my self-confidence diminishing?

1. When taking on a new task. Right now, for me that means learning to swim again after not having done so for many years.

2. Being introduced to a man who is dating someone younger and better looking than I am.

3. Playing bridge with experts.

Create your own list.

I've talked about how the world is a confusing place with the jumble of conflicting messages and demands that each of us faces. Now I'm going to present you with the real secret to breaking the hold of that confusion. It may sound simple, but if it were, wouldn't you be doing it instead of reading about it?

The world "out there" isn't going to change no matter how fervently you wish or pray. But "your world," where you do have some influence, can change to reflect your preferences in the same way that your cupboards and refrigerator reflect your shopping and eating preferences. Here is how to get started.

Ask yourself where and when you feel your best. Then write down what makes you feel good about yourself — what works for you, not for your friends, but for you. From baking blueberry muffins for a neighbor, walking in the rain, arranging flowers, to a simple bike ride to nowhere in particular because it reminds you of your childhood. You can work on expanding your list of what you enjoy doing or feeling about yourself as long as none of the items listed hurts others.

After making your list, decide what is stopping you from doing the things that make you feel good. Right then, assertively decide to start doing some of the things that make you feel good. Remember, the only person with the right answer for you, is YOU.

Your happiness, confidence, motivation, and assertive skills all depend on finding the experiences that give you pleasure. If health is a priority, what is stopping you from doing what it takes? Only yourself.

Let's begin with freeing yourself from the "stinking thinking" that stops you from doing the things you need to do to reach a goal. But keep it simple. Avoid complicating the issue by thinking you will have everything on your terms tomorrow afternoon by 2:30.

Review your list about what you enjoy and, while you're at it, list all the things you dislike. However, try not to be unreasonable. For example, if you like how it feels to lose weight but dislike doing what you need to do to lose it, the answer is, "Tough!" Check your grandiosity at the door and realize that IT JUST WON'T HAPPEN WITHOUT THE NECESSARY COMMITMENT AND SACRIFICES. I adore acting. But I am not going to kid myself; I lack training and the desire to go for training. So making acting a goal would be unreasonable. However, I can compromise and join a play reading group. Ask your friends where they think you "shine." This may help you gain insights about yourself that will help you make decisions about future goals.

Challenge the negative head talk that adults are notorious for because it undermines your chances for developing more self-confidence. Force yourself to think about your pluses. In situations where you lack confidence, it's OK to bluff or pretend. When you pretend long enough you will begin living up to your pretenses.

A Review: Assertiveness, Change, and Risk Taking

Five reasons why people act non-assertively or passively:

1. Failure to distinguish assertion from aggression
2. Believing that acting non-assertively is polite or considerate. They may have been taught:
   a. that it is impolite to interrupt even if the other person talks *ad nauseam.*
   b. not to disagree with someone who is older, disabled, or has higher status.
   c. not to refuse food at someone's home.
   d. to deflect any compliment.
3. Failure to accept personal rights. That means they feel they do not have the right to their own emotions. Often they believe that they shouldn't have these feelings in the first place.
4. Belief that one's non-assertion will actually help somebody.
5. Anxiety about negative consequences:

   "I will lose affection and approval."

   "Others will think I am foolish or selfish."

   "I will hurt someone's feelings, or they will reject me."

Speaking up about issues you feel strongly about is, for many, the most difficult task they face, and yet IT IS THE MOST REWARDING.

It is difficult to tell people things they don't want to hear. It is much easier to "go along." But what happens to your soul when you repeatedly deny yourself the right and opportunity to speak your mind? Remaining silent when you feel strongly about an issue is bound to make you feel rotten about yourself.

When the time comes to express your thoughts, don't just think about it — JUST DO IT.

Waiting for the perfect time won't work. It may never come. Your goal is not to devise a "perfect solution." Rather it is to behave assertively with style. Acting assertively with style simply means speaking up when speaking up makes sense — when it is appropriate, always considering the consequences, and being sensitive about not sounding aggressive. Understand clearly how you come across to others. It's not an easy assignment. It takes a lot of awareness and practice, which you can do if you start at the beginning with realistic expectations.

Your REBT skills will guide you into assertiveness that is authoritative, polite, and dignified while showing respect for others. Being assertive is the most important tool to help you make life happen instead of waiting for it to happen to you.

If you have bought into the Rational Thinking component of this program and you find that you still are not doing the things you want to do, then you need to accept that your negative head talk is stronger than your new, assertive, rational head talk. Example: *"I know I should be making an eating chart, but somehow I continue to procrastinate and tell myself over and over again I'll do it."* A better message is, *"Though I don't feel like keeping an eating chart, I have to do it in order to gain control over my eating habits. If I fail, I will have to accept the consequence,"* like not buying the dress you had promised yourself as a reward for keeping the chart.

What if you find that you are not keeping the eating chart and you go ahead and buy the dress? Then it would be smart to give up at this time, because your actions send the message: you don't want it enough. Stop playing games and boring others. It is important to understand that IT IS OKAY TO NOT WANT IT. It is your body, your life, your decision.

Living Thin is for people who want to be in the game. For those people the road is full of obstacles, but they are up to the challenge. They "do it" even though they "don't feel like doing it." They are able to push themselves, practice skills, and congratulate themselves for their successes while not giving up when they goof. In their quest to Live Thin and Healthily, they use assertion skills to stay on course. They speak to others and themselves with vigor and force in order to free themselves from neurotic behaviors such as self-deception and denial. The clearest and most common neurosis in the game of losing weight is the one where you insist you want to lose weight but, at the same time, refuse to do anything about it.

Perhaps the most important questions you need to face before even thinking about change is 1) will you be able to deal with the consequences of failing to make small changes, and 2) will you be able to withstand the negative responses that others will have to your being assertive?

If you are going to fall apart when others notice you are changing and taking charge of your own issues on your terms, you will go back to your old habits. You see the cycle, the pattern, of how unassertive people wind up being defined by others?

BUT YOU DO HAVE A CHOICE — return to old ways or accept that their upsettedness at your changing IS THEIR PROBLEM NOT YOURS!

Example 1: Some years ago Dr. Marian Robinson, former head of speech and drama at Goucher College in Towson, Maryland, told me that she was working with a young student who had a lateral lisp that produced a whistling sound when she spoke. The two of them worked for many hours on eradicating this very unattractive lisp, because when you hear someone with this particular disability, you don't really hear what they are saying, you only hear the whistle.

The girl went home for a holiday visit. When she returned, she knocked on Dr. Robinson's door and spoke with her old lisp. Dr. Robinson said, "Child, what happened?" The student went on to relate that at home her friends were astonished at the change in her speech and complained bitterly that this was not the Gloria they remembered. They were uncomfortable around the new Gloria. Gloria returned to her lisp so they would feel more comfortable.

Gloria asked Dr. Robinson for more help. Dr. Robinson said, "Absolutely not." Why did she refuse? Because she was unwilling to waste her time on someone who did not have the stamina to assert her own needs.

Example 2: During an Adventures in Learning course on assertiveness training that I designed, a group of women complained about a friend who was in the course. They had been friends with Marilyn for years and she had been so passive, such a pussycat. And now she was anything but! They saw no advantage in her taking the course. What they were saying was that she had become as assertive as they were. They had lost their servant and she had gained her soul. Can we blame them for being upset?

Remembering who is in charge puts you in charge. Even if you are in a situation where someone else is the boss, you do not relinquish control of your feelings, desires, and needs.

A simple method for being in charge of what you are attempting to communicate is to remember to pause between sentences. It gives you a chance to think and be in control of what you will say next.

To become an assertive individual you first have to know yourself. Being assertive is a personal experience. However, it is not the answer to each and every problem. The more you know about yourself and the more adept you become at identifying how assertion can help you personally, the easier it will be to assert yourself with style — in other words to develop "presence."

Very often you and I hear people say that so and so has "presence." This person has an assurance, a confidence, that communicates itself to others. This person is communicating, "I know who I am, I have an inner strength, I often think before I speak," or more subtly, "I am able to distance myself from situations while remaining involved."

SUMMARY

The good and bad news about change:

The real battle is in my head. The good news is that I have what it takes to speak up — whenever I CHOOSE to do so. More good news is that I can THINK myself into feeling any way I want to think by forcing myself to THINK with AUTHORITY — with VIGOR. I know that my response to what I am saying will be dictated mainly by the degree of authority I use when I talk to myself.

The bad news is that changing a habit developed over a lifetime will take time — and SO WHAT? Also, I will try and fail at times, but that's OK.

If you fail to "speak up," SO WHAT? The next time, or the time after, I promise, you will become as assertive as you care to be and excel if you refuse to give up on yourself. Enjoy your journey into the magical world of asserting yourself, but also remember to avoid overdoing — and always think of the consequences.

8

Getting Started

Dealing With Not Having Enough Time

How many times have you heard the comment, "I have a few hours to kill"? Why would anyone want to "kill time?" Time is elusive and easy to ignore, but once it's gone, it's gone.

You can recapture a lost relationship, but once your time has run out, there is no bringing it back.

"No time to think about food."

"No time to think about exercise."

"No time to even think about practicing assertiveness skills or the art of rational thinking to avoid undue stress."

If that sounds like you, I want you to give some thought to time itself. Think about the many hours poor health requires: going to doctors, missing work, convalescing, and just feeling bad for days or weeks at a time.

Here are a few practical suggestions for handling time and hunger:

1. Have snacks on hand that you can turn to easily without much preparation so you can eat in the car if you need to (carrot/celery sticks, apples, a healthy sandwich with a slice of cheese and lightly dressed). You can also travel with a coffee thermos so you can sit and read the morning paper. But let's not read and drive at the same time!

2. Avoid skipping meals, especially breakfast. Skipping breakfast slows down your metabolism. Eating breakfast perks it up.

3. Instead of eating heavy meals, try eating frequently with a calorie control plan to guide you. This approach is called "grazing." By grazing, you will avoid large meals, which tend to overwhelm your body with calories that it cannot metabolize at that moment.

4. Remember, it is not how often you eat, but what you are eating and how many calories you are consuming that matters.

Dealing With Eating Out

Many women and men have decided that eating out is better than eating in — so much so, in fact, that it has become a regular part of accepted eating patterns. To handle eating out, you need to have specific guidelines so you can know in advance that you will not destroy your best-laid plans.

First, your attitude about eating out, regardless of how expensive or inexpensive the restaurant: The staff is there to please you. They want you to have a good time and to return. Be assertive about stating your wishes and needs. You do not need the approval of your server. And don't be so sure your friends will think you aggressive if you speak up and ask for what you want.

Next, develop the habit of deciding approximately what you want before you go and how to handle the "free extras," beginning with the rolls that often greet you on your table. Unless you and your partner are opposed to the idea, I suggest you ask your server to "hold the rolls," garlic bread, or whatever. You may tell your server that you intend to have the roll with a bit of butter or jelly as a dessert.

Here are a few other suggestions:

1. Request all your sauces and dressings "on the side." This way, you can control your portions. I like to "dilute" my rich dressings by adding water and then spooning it onto my food. This makes "less go further."

2. Choose whole grain bread whenever possible.

3. Avoid fried foods. Lightly sautéed foods are fine.

4. Order a baked potato instead of French fries (fried in oil) or mashed (butter is added in the kitchen).

5. Return food that you do not find satisfactory.

6. Do not be bashful about taking home the portion you have not eaten. This has become quite "stylish" and is very intelligent. Ask for a doggie bag. This way you won't be tempted to eat everything on your plate.

7. When starting a new eating plan, feel free to bring your own dressing. Remember, most dressings cost about 100–200 calories per teaspoon.

8. Expect special service. You are the guest and are paying for everything. When you expect it and request it, you are simply asserting your "diner's rights." When you do so, the chances of complaining when it's over are almost nil. The chances of enjoying yourself are greatly increased.

9. Where you eat has much to do with what you will eat. When deciding where you will eat, assert your preferences to companions and force yourself to consider the consequences of your choice if you are eating alone.

10. Think about health rather than how much your meal costs in terms of what you may leave on your plate. OVEREATING IS NEVER A BARGAIN.

11. Most restaurants have meals that are not high in calories. Think in terms of chicken and fish broiled and lightly seasoned. (Read and reread sections on how easy it is to add hidden calories and about how easy it is to omit them without spoiling a first-class meal).

12. Consider making a meal from: clear soup, one appetizer, a salad, a roll with jelly or a half pat of butter and coffee.

13. At salad bars, watch out for the dressings. One ladle can cost you approximately 200 calories.

14. Have a drink, but watch the calories. One wine spritzer equals 80 calories. One vodka collins has 180. One Perrier with a twist of lemon has NO CALORIES.

15. Check Getting Started list in Chapter 4 for additional ideas.

Living Thin Works!

As a student of Living Thin you can lose weight healthily and forever without giving up your favorite foods, and you can be in charge of your daily stress. You can actually become your own nutritionist and your own therapist. Talk about self-esteem and being a role model for others!

Weight problems are not curable, only controllable. I urge you not to discuss the issue with your naturally slender friends. They haven't a clue about the problems and challenges we face. Over the years I would, on occasion, invite a slender friend (who had never had to battle with controlling weight) to assist me with the program. These people taught me very soon that our problems simply fail to register for them. These issues are abstractions to them, nothing more.

When you "goof up" on occasion, and I promise you will, all you need to do is whip out your eating chart, place it on the fridge in the kitchen, begin the same principles, and I guarantee you will be back on track almost immediately. There is something magical about keeping the chart. It's so simple. You're starting a journey that will keep you and your body operating at peak level.

CREATING THE PERMANENT CONNECTION

After teaching my program for many years, a message emerged loud and clear. I received praise from most participants who had discovered newfound commitment, motivation, assertiveness, knowledge and success at becoming slender.

Because weight loss requires constant attention, I began offering successful graduates a program called the PERMANENT CONNECTION. Its goal was to provide time for more work and practice. Participating in the Permanent Connection is a splendid way for people who want to Live Thin to become more secure in their efforts and skills. It works wonders by reinforcing the information and techniques we deal with in class.

I see no reason why my readers cannot form their own Permanent Connection groups. Here is how to get it started.

Invite three or more (as many as 20) people to participate. The number is less important compared to the quality of how the program is conducted. There are two conditions that need to be fulfilled for the Permanent Connection to work. One is to have a leader. It may not be easy finding the right person, but it won't work unless you do. The leader is required to have the problem AND know what tough love is about, i.e., caring enough for each member to enforce the rules laid down by the group. It is about accountability. That means honoring meeting dates and times regardless of inconvenience and seeing to it that the second condition is implemented — the contract.

At meetings, each member is weighed in, and the leader's assistant is available to go over the chart of a member who has failed to fulfill the contract terms she agreed to when she joined the group. The terms of the contract need to be realistic (no sense in promising to lose 10 pounds a week or exercising 60 minutes a day if you've been inactive for 20 years), and the penalty for failing has to be severe enough, be painful, or at least very uncomfortable. Otherwise members will have no incentive to succeed. When I was teaching full time, there was a contract for the Living Thin class. Failure to live up to the contract lost the student their tuition, and they were asked to leave the class. If members of your group say "that's too much money," that is a good place to set the penalty. Remember, there is an easy way to avoid being penalized — do the things you need to do. It is very important to discuss all these issues in front of the participants of the Permanent Connection to provide a clear, collective understanding of the rules.

Several years ago, I began teaching at a school in Florida where the director of education insisted that I omit the contract from the class or at least the part about asking students to leave the class. Though I don't recall any students leaving, I do recall having the lowest success rate of any class I had ever conducted. There is no way I would consider ever teaching or recommending a support group without the contract being required. This limits the program to people who have the courage to follow through. I attribute the huge success I have had with my program for so many years to both the content and to the student's knowing that I would, indeed, enforce this contract.

9

Nuts, Bolts, and "Staying Tuned"

Why Diets Often Fail — Especially for Busy People

"No matter what I read or hear, I still wish I could go to sleep and wake up thin." Sorry, if you have even minimal awareness of the past and current state of the weight loss story, you know there is no magic.

Entrepreneurs are sensitive to the time demands on all of us. In the weight loss game, they exploit the overweight person's quick-fix mentality. The problem is, you are not learning how to deal with the REAL WORLD — eating out, socializing, traveling, time demands, stress of daily life, disappointments, anger, and much more.

Any idea that emphasizes a temporary approach, such as pills or milk shakes, can never succeed on a permanent basis and may often have harmful side effects. Likewise, any program that "tells" you all you need to know about weight loss and then proceeds to pay its rent by selling you food is designed to make you financially (and psychologically) dependent on the program.

Food, Food, Everywhere — Haven't Lost a Pound

FOOD — What will I eat for breakfast, lunch, and dinner? For overweights the topic of eating is a complex issue, one that is intimately connected to the way you live. For overweights, life is like a carnival midway with food as the attraction on all sides.

Food issues permeate our lives from the cradle to the grave. From birthdays to wakes we are eating every day. Most of us are thinking about it hourly: *"What will I eat; with whom will I eat, or with whom I will not eat; where will I eat?"*

It used to be we didn't have the information we needed to make wise food choices. The problem now is that we have too much information, and since so much of it is contradictory, the average person often walks away from what may have become a serious problem in his or her life. Some of this information is very good, however, and walking away is never a good solution. THE SOLUTION IS TO BECOME YOUR OWN NUTRI-TIONIST. Read. Think. Learn as you grow. But meanwhile, stay with the Living Thin and Living Young basics so that you can lose weight and achieve better health — mentally and phys-ically — while you continue to educate yourself.

EXERCISE

We agree that healthy heads promote healthy behaviors. In turn, your attitude about your health and the aging process will de-termine whether you are willing to involve yourself in the activi-ties necessary for creating a healthy lifestyle — such as exercise.

You may say, "Why bother?" Personally, I exercise because I care about *me*. I find reasons to move more because each day I engage in physical activity I find myself eating a little more healthily that same day. And I find I have a difficult time holding onto my depression when I exercise. Exercise and depression simply seem to be incompatible.

I find that I can eat more and weigh less on days I exercise. Best of all, I find I feel better when I exercise, and the better I feel, the less upset I am about everything. Exercising depresses my appetite. The more I move, the more satisfied I seem to be with smaller portions. I've learned that getting upset is easier when I am sluggish.

These insights motivate me to find some time for some exercise every day. It can be as little as ten minutes, but it has to be a priority.

There is plenty in your head about why you can't exercise or why you gave up exercising. You may say, "I know exercise could help me lose weight and it's better for my knees, back, and head, but, unfortunately, I do not have the time." Or, "I know I need to exercise for my heart, my hypertension, and to stave off arthritis (or to get relief from it), but I can't seem to get started and I simply don't have the time." Or, everyone's favorite, "I find exercise boring."

In response to these excuses, I am telling you that finding a simple formula for daily exercise is not TOO hard, it's just hard. And so what if it is? I suggest you think real hard about all the things you manage to find time for (TV, movies, socializing, eating) and realize that you are constantly making choices and constantly finding the time to carry out these choices.

Exercise may be boring, but being overweight and deliberately inviting health problems is boring too. So we are back to making choices. I suggest you think hard about the consequences of your decision not to exercise, and always remember, YOU DON'T ALWAYS HAVE TO FEEL LIKE IT, YOU JUST HAVE TO DO IT. Do you want to be healthy? The choice is yours.

The medical literature is filled with information on children and adults who are in harm's way simply as a result of their failure to exercise. One study shows that obese men have a 33 percent greater risk of dying from any type of cancer than do average-weight men. Obese women have a 55 percent greater risk of dying from cancer than do average-weight women.

Dr. John Foreyt, director of The Behavioral Modification Research Center at Baylor University of Medicine, has suggested that public policy be changed to allow people exercise opportunities at work and at school.

What a sad commentary on our society — that we as individuals are not mature enough to do it for ourselves! The result? Just what we see today: too many people getting too fat, becoming sick as a result, needing medical care for conditions that are preventable yet still costs everyone (the sick and the well, the fat and the slender) more and more; and higher incidence of diseases that we'd all rather live without.

If you have avoided exercise for longer than you care to admit, also avoid overdoing it when you begin. Select one form of movement, jogging in place or on a trampoline, doing "the bicycle" on your back — legs in the air, walking vigorously or merely swinging your arms while you do a "heel to toe" movement with your feet. Adopt this form of exercise or try a variety, but get in the habit even if it is only a few minutes at a time.

Slow is better than fast when you are getting started. It lasts longer. You can feel great about yourself without giving up a moment of your other activities. Do your jogging in place, skipping rope, or a series of stretching exercises first thing in the morning. Refuse to start your day without at least three minutes of concentrated movement. Don't minimize the value of starting modestly because BEING IN THE HABIT OF EXERCISING IS MORE IMPORTANT THAN WHAT EXERCISE YOU DO OR EVEN HOW LONG YOU DO IT.

Think about and look for opportunities to fit in simple movements such as taking the stairs instead of the elevator, parking your car at a distance from the store, or taking a walk at the mall. You may enjoy finding a buddy, or you may prefer going it alone. Take a walk during a lunch break. Think about moving more and sitting less. And remember to talk to your doctor before you start to exercise.

The more exercise the better, and a little is better than none. Any kind of movement is better than no kind of movement. SO GET MOVING!

"I know what to do, so why don't I do it?

I don't do it because I don't feel like doing it."

ATTITUDES AND BEHAVIORS

Students of Living Thin become practitioners of Rational Emotive Behavior Therapy, which is all about attitudes. The essence of rational thinking is that there is no way you can control the behavior of other people. But *you* are the captain of your emotional ship. The way you respond is *entirely* up to you.

> Don't expect
> motivation to
> fall from the
> sky. It rises up
> from the grit.

The following statements briefly summarize the Living Thin philosophy on several major points on which you may need to work. Dog-ear this page. Come back to it when you're feeling weak and need a quick shot of motivation. Be sure to leave in the self-esteem that comes from doing hard things.

MOTIVATION

Motivation is the key, and you may be surprised to learn that you already have it. The fact that you're reading this proves you have motivation! What you need is the head talk that motivates you to use your motivation. For example, I refuse to cave in to the negative feelings like boredom, loneliness, depression, and fatigue that destroy my motivation. There is no way you're going to find the motivation to do hard things when you're exhausted. You can't say no to a cookie or an extra portion when you are lonely, bored, or depressed. The answer lies in talking to yourself, making yourself aware of the feelings that erode your motivation. If I'm exhausted and I know that my motivation dies when I'm exhausted, I'm going to stay away from food at those times. Accept the fact that only when you are willing to resolve these issues will you be able to do the things you want to do. You will love the results, especially the self-esteem that comes from doing hard things.

Low Frustration Tolerance. LFT involves an absolute horror at feeling any form of discomfort about any issue related to weight loss. You may have the message in your head that "when I am under stress, I simply cannot say 'no' to food and I find it impossible to do any exercise. It's just too hard."

The solution is to concentrate on substituting the following statements.

"While I find it difficult to say 'no,' I am convinced that failing to say 'no' is harder because I am not willing to live with the consequences." And, *"As long as I am working on a lifestyle that is moderately satisfying, I am willing to do it gradually, even in the face of daily stresses."*

Self-Downing. Even though you may have failed in the past, you can learn to live healthily and enjoy it! Each day is just that — a new start, another opportunity to get what you want for yourself, to succeed. Don't listen to the voice inside your head that says, *"I have tried over and over to lose weight and even when I do lose it, it comes back again. This proves I lack the self-control to make it. Why bother?"*

The solution is that the only thing you've proved is that diets can't work. Now that you've educated yourself and discovered via *doing*, not just reading the Living Thin message, you are learning that you DO have the self-control. It's the lack of education that leads you to think you had no self-control.

Self-Acceptance. You are a valuable addition to the human race You are unique. Never forget it. Of course you have foibles. We all do and So What! Accepting yourself unconditionally means fully accepting yourself with both good and bad behaviors. Don't allow yourself to think, "I've failed to keep my weight under control. I am a bad person."

The solution is to avoid making unrealistic demands. By following the Living Thin philosophy (approximating caloric intake, keeping an eating chart, engaging in some physical activity), you are learning roughly how much you can eat and how much you may have to exercise in order to lose or maintain your weight.

In other words, you will find a personal prescription for healthy and permanent weight loss. After learning to accept the information about your body (which differs for each of us) you will be armed with indisputable data that will allow you to make personal choices about your goals. At this point you MAY be willing to settle for a size 12 instead of a size 6. Isn't that great?

The most important part of this experience is ACCEPTING YOURSELF AND THE WAY YOUR BODY WORKS. When I'm asked to explain my program, my response is that it's a different program for each person. What an individual gets out of the program depends on what she brings to it and what she needs from it.

How I Learned to Accept My Compulsive Nature

I love my Living Thin Program. In addition to teaching me **how to eat** rather than how to diet, it taught me how to accept my nature, for better and for worse. I am a compulsive personality. I was born that way, and I plan on dying that way. There is no way I even want to change my compulsiveness — but I can still Live Thin because I've learned to work around my compulsiveness. I know in my heart of hearts, just as you do in yours, that eating a delicious piece of cake on an empty stomach is acceptable only if I allow myself to goof off and go for six or seven slices and enjoy it knowing I'll probably gain a pound. But if it is that delicious and I enjoy it that much, it's worth every calorie and I don't have to feel guilty. Why not? Because I have educated myself about how to handle it. Living Thin has provided the intelligent solution.

I don't have to give up all my favorite foods. I can still have my bagels and my cocktails. It's all a matter of what I can and cannot afford. This knowledge allows me to make choices that make Living Thin easy because I don't have to feel deprived. All I am really giving up are foods I don't care that much about anyway. In the past I ate just to eat. I am now giving more thought to my choices and find that I am enjoying my food more and eating less and that there is more quality than quantity in my food choices these days as health has become an overriding issue.

Because I don't have to be perfect, I can relax about any and all choices. The thinking behind my program is pretty much the same thinking you might have about the car you drive or the home you elect to live in — it's about choices and what you can afford. Only you can make choices that will work for you — a grown-up you, who realizes that not feeling deprived is not the same as always getting exactly what you want every moment. Living Thin is about having it all, but not all the time.

Living Thin is about accepting who you are, assuming responsibility for yourself and finally, it's about growing up — whatever your age. That is why the theme of Living Thin is BECOMING YOUR OWN NUTRITIONIST AND YOUR OWN THERAPIST.

We are living in a society that endorses the belief, the hoax, that there is someone out there that can do it for you. The truth is that you have all the answers within yourself, in your head. You have the will and the desire and when you find the answers that will work for you, you will have found the key to your success.

That involves getting your head screwed on straight. Then the rest will follow. You will then be able to be comfortable and motivated to do the things you know how to do, but in many instances, are not doing.

WHAT IS GOOD EMOTIONAL HEALTH?

Becoming emotionally healthy means becoming a non-neurotic healthy human being. This is not something that falls from the sky. You can't depend on pills, magic, or programs. The only person who can help you build emotional muscle is yourself.

Expect some setbacks. Understanding the information you are reading now will not automatically give you healthy eating and living habits or cause all your "upsettedness" to be resolved immediately.

During the many years I have taught Living Thin, participants would leave class determined to do whatever needed to be done. But without a weekly phone call they would revert to their old habits. Why? Because you have a tendency to forget, to not pay such close attention after a few days. When you're not reminded, other priorities get in the way. As you read this material, or if you talk about it (a wonderful method for reinforcing the message while it is still in your head), doing it becomes less difficult.

As you read this material you feel motivated to whip out an eating chart. You make a plan and the first few days are fairly easy. Within a few days you discover how easy it is to feel satisfied to lose weight. It all seems so simple. But along the way you stop doing it. Why?

Because your priorities get shuffled. Life happens. A wonderful solution to avoid this is to get other people involved. Helping others is an ideal way to reinforce what you yourself want to learn and make part of your routine. Practice this rational therapy on others. As you help them, you will hear yourself making rational statements you need to use yourself, every day. In this way you are constantly "reselling" rational thinking to yourself. Restating these messages will make your rational thinking skills stronger.

Do not blame yourself for slipping back. It is natural to regress. Expect to go backwards at times, but refuse to get upset. Refuse to give up. When you have a backup plan you don't have to get upset, because you know failure is not inevitable. Suppose you've slipped and gained a pound or two in a day. Just place that eating chart on your fridge, and guess what, you've got it made. You can get yourself back on track.

But you must respect the chart and the process. It's not the chart, it's your attitude about the chart. If you respect the chart, honor it, you can't lose (or should I say you can't help BUT lose). It will serve you well. The chart becomes your policeman, which is what you need. With the eating chart you can't chicken out when you do poorly.

It's the same with your emotions. You will not be perfect in responding to others. At times you will become angrier or more anxious, depressed, or guilty than you want to become. As a human being these emotions are natural. You wouldn't want to become a flatliner emotionally. Don't be alarmed or upset with yourself if, on occasion, you overreact to something somebody did or said. Slipping back into your old way of thinking is to be expected at times. It's bound to happen. But it's the way you handle these slips that counts. Remember, everyone has fumbled. It's the recovery that counts.

The essence of sound mental and emotional health is summed up in The Serenity Prayer, attributed to Friedrich Oetinger and Reinhold Niebuhr.

> God grant me the serenity to accept the things I cannot change, courage to change the things I can, and the wisdom to know the difference.

Think about how ridiculous it is to become enraged when a souped-up teenager is tailgating you. Why not simply wave him on? He has the right to drive dangerously. We hope he receives his comeuppance, but in the meantime, let him go.

The person who wins at life is the one who refuses to give up, refuses to feel rejected or down when life rains on his parade. What kind of person do you want to be? The choice is yours.

It could take years to become really good at Living Thin. So What? How long does it take to become a good golfer or pianist? How long to master a language? Learning about yourself and learning to break old habits and developing new ones is a complicated process, and it takes time. Give yourself the time.

When you slip, don't be surprised. You know what to do to get back on track. If you've gained weight, get out the eating chart. If you notice yourself feeling depressed, begin working vigorously on your REBT skills and avoid "shoulding" on yourself. Force yourself to make plans and follow through on them. Sure it's hard, but it's not too hard. It will be harder if you give up.

When you are disturbed, ask yourself, "What am I telling myself that is causing my upsettedness? What ideas am I holding that I can challenge?" Then, forcefully dispute these irrational ideas. It inevitably works to lessen your degree of upsettedness.

Finding Your Own Answers

No two people's heads are alike. That's the good news. The rest of the news is that each person needs to find his own answers. Because there is no one just like you, each person needs to take personal responsibility for finding solutions to his or her complex problems.

By following the guidelines at the end of this chapter, you will find out, within a week or two at the most, how much you can eat and exercise without feeling deprived of your favorite foods to lose weight gradually and permanently. Additionally, you will be on your way to creating a lifestyle of eating and moving that works for you and that you can comfortably practice for the rest of your life.

I designed my program based on my realization that looking for answers from someone else — looking for someone else to take care of *my business* — was NEVER GOING TO WORK! (Reread Chapter 1 to understand why diets won't ever work). I realized early that though there are many ways of taking it off, keeping it off is the answer to permanent weight loss. The choices you make for keeping it off need to be compatible with your tastes, values, and preferences — in other words — WITH YOU! What works for Harriet won't necessarily work for Henrietta. The program that works for everyone, works for no one.

DOING IT WITH SELF-DISCIPLINE
(It's Not A Dirty Word)

Mary Lou walks around depressed much of the time. Her problem is not physiological but psychological. When you examine her history and background, you can see the causes for most of her problems. Not all, but many, are rooted in her refusal to exercise the Art of Discipline. The art of discipline is one of the most powerful phrases in our language.

Mary Lou needs to lose weight. She suffers from high blood pressure and high cholesterol, and she has weakness in her knees from carrying too much weight. Despite what her doctor recommends, she cannot motivate herself to do the things she needs to do. In other words, her root problem is a lack of discipline! SHE

> You don't have
> to FEEL like
> doing it. You just
> have to do it.

WANTS TO LOSE WEIGHT BUT DOESN'T WANT IT ENOUGH TO DO WHAT SHE NEEDS TO DO.

How can Mary Lou make herself do the things she needs to do? How can she find the self-discipline that is missing? No wonder she is depressed.

Mary Lou has the same problem in other areas of her life. She would love to learn to play golf for social reasons. She is sure she'd enjoy the activity, but again lacks the discipline. Others call it "will." I say she doesn't want to do the things that would move her toward her goals because SHE DOESN'T FEEL LIKE DOING THEM.

What it takes for Mary Lou — you, me and all the rest of us — is the self-discipline to do hard things. It is easy to get yourself to do things you feel like doing, but making yourself do the things you don't feel like doing is another matter. Without developing this skill you cannot reach any goal, whatever that goal may be.

Your level of discipline will determine your success in any and all areas of your life. Here is an excellent example. Two high school students, Henry and John, both dream of going on to important careers, but Henry resents studying for his exams. Instead of studying he chooses to join his friends at the movie theater. You might say, "Well, he is young. I don't blame him." John, on the other hand, also finds studying for his exams boring and would rather turn in early or go see a film, but he toughs it out because he has decided that avoiding the studying will create other problems. HE IS SO RIGHT! Henry will pay a big price for catering to his need for immediate gratification.

Apply this scenario to people who are overweight, and you will find that most overweights find excuses to overeat and say that it will be easier tomorrow. WRONG! It will be harder tomorrow. As difficult as it is, it is nevertheless easier now.

A major cause of poor discipline is the way you choose to talk to yourself. *"If I could find an easy way, why not?"* There is nothing wrong with finding an easy way. The problem is, there are no easy answers. However, there is a simple solution. GROW UP AND EDUCATE YOURSELF. MAKE YOUR OWN CHOICES. Live Thin.

Your choices, whatever they are, have a thousand percent more chance of succeeding than the best choice another person makes for you. To work, the answer has to come from you. It is the easy way to get the job done. By thinking about calories (how much you can consume) and exercise (how much you can realistically start doing), you can make a decision that suits you, that will work for you.

> Even if you are on
> the right track,
> You'll get run over if
> you just sit there.
>
> — Will Rogers

Soon you will realize that you can have the best of all worlds: food you enjoy, weight loss, more energy, and no deprivation. As you learn your Living Thin skills and put them into practice, you will feel satisfied with your choices and the practice becomes easier. Eventually, it becomes a lifestyle.

You can develop the habit of becoming a disciplined person yourself. Each time you force yourself to do what you need to do, the next time becomes easier. Refuse to dump on yourself when you goof. Refusing to give up is the magic that makes it work.

THE CHALLENGE OF CHANGE

The Good News and the Bad News

Good news first. Some typical comments from Living Thin students:

- *I really feel good about the changes I am introducing in my life via my Living Thin education*

- *I'm not only eating healthier foods but delicious ones*

- *I find I am feeling so much better physically. I have more energy and less aches and pains*

- *Emotionally, I am astonishing even myself. I no longer get upset over the small stuff — slow traffic, mail that doesn't arrive, etc.*

- *I think I am becoming a philosopher and find that I am willing to do some — not all — of the things I've been told about being in charge, like planning daily meals, refusing to feel guilty when I goof. Wow, what a difference. What bliss*

- *I feel that I've freed myself from a lot of garbage*

- *I am losing weight finally and wouldn't dream of returning to my old habits. How can I be so sure? Because I'd feel like a fool giving up the health I've picked up along the way*

- *When I began, my goal was weight loss only. That alone no longer satisfies me*

- *Though I am delighted with my weight loss, I'm even more excited about my newfound emotional and physical health*

Now for the Bad News:

"My friends, relatives and enemies (especially my enemies) are having a hard time with their new view of me. They need to change the former image they have of me, which makes them feel uncomfortable. They are much more concerned with the discomfort 'my new me' gives them, than with the improvements I've won for myself. They even resent the changes. THEY certainly don't need them or want them. So much for human nature . . . and yet I understand their dilemma."

The BEST News — Try telling yourself this:

Change is tough for everyone — those viewing it and those doing it. However, there is absolutely no way I am going to allow myself to slide backwards. They have a perfect right to be upset and I in turn have the same rights.

I am practicing a new theory for myself: no one can upset me without my permission or make me feel guilty. Others are responsible for their own upsettedness, and in time, if I hold fast, which I have every intention of doing, these same people will grow accustomed to the new me and begin respecting and admiring me. I will probably become a role model for them. That takes time, but I've become disciplined enough to be able to wait, and I've learned a lot about how to get the junk out of my head.

The Art of Talking to Yourself

A powerful tool for motivating and disciplining yourself to do what you need to do is the art of talking to yourself.

Whether we are aware of it or not, there is a continual dialogue going on within ourselves. This internal dialogue all too often contains pessimistic messages: *"I'm so clumsy." "I never have enough time to exercise." "I am always saying the wrong thing."* According to Dr. John Ingram Walker, a clinical professor of psychiatry at the University of Texas Health Science Center and director of Education at Laurel Ridge Hospital in San Antonio, "It is natural to think negatively because of the negative messages we read and listen to in newspapers, TV, and radio daily. We need to train ourselves to think in a positive fashion."

"Stinking Thinking"

What are you telling yourself that may not be positive and/or rational? Are you guilty of any of the following categories of self-talk?

1. **All or Nothing Thinking** — It's perfection or nothing for you. "If I don't go to my daughter's play, I'M A FAILURE as a mother. If I eat this candy bar, I'VE FAILED at this diet."

2. **Generalization** — It's all or nothing for you. "I've gained three pounds. I'll NEVER lose ANY weight."

3. **Jumping to Conclusions** — You think you know all, see all, even the future, and your conclusions are often negative. "He didn't call me back. I'll NEVER find a partner!"

4. **Awfulizing** — To put it simply, you exaggerate! No one but you ever has a problem. "If I have to wear a size 14 dress, IT WILL KILL ME!"

5. **Shoulding on yourself** — You put yourself on guilt trips. "I should, I ought to, I must." And when you can't attain perfection, you give up. See number one!

Mind-Body Reactions to Negative Self-Talk

These negative messages create feelings of guilt, hopelessness, helplessness, anxiety, and depression. Putting yourself down and blowing problems out of proportion will not only have negative effects on your self-esteem and emotional state, but can burden your body as well.

Psychologists and psychiatrists believe that "negative thinkers" are more apt to stress related headaches, stomach upsets, high blood pressure, and depression. The stress from such negative thinking can create an additional set of problems by forming a vicious cycle where thinking becomes more and more polarized and distorted.

Under this type of stress, it becomes nearly impossible to think clearly or take appropriate action in the case of a real emergency.

What can you do to break the cycle?

Learn the art of self-talk!

Develop an awareness of the connection between your thoughts and feelings. As you experience an emotion, identify it as: depression, anger, guilt, frustration, or anxiety. Understand the shadings of these emotional states:

1. DEPRESSION — blue, down, low

2. ANGER — furious, enraged

3. GUILT — shame, embarrassed

4. FRUSTRATION — disappointed, discontented

5. ANXIETY — fearful, scared, nervous, uneasy

The goal of rational thinking is to reduce, diffuse, or at times erase negative feelings. This is not to rid you of your emotions but rather to relieve the extreme unhealthy emotions. Feeling low is one thing; feeling depressed is another. When you lose control of your emotional response, you are no longer in total control of your behavior, and all too often the results can be disastrous. All too often this loss of control leads to your saying and doing things you would never dream of doing or saying had you been in control.

Another danger is overreacting. It leads to overeating. Let's assume I find myself consuming two bagels instead of the one I had planned on having, an easy error for me. As you know, I am passionate about bagels. If I dismiss my eating more with a "So What!" I will probably be left only with some regret and a plan to somehow make up for the approximately 350 calories I hadn't planned on. But if I allow my error to upset me, I can easily begin experiencing guilt which in turn leads to overeating.

The key is training myself to respond intelligently, thinking my way through the situation **rationally** rather than irrationally.

Using Positive Statements

Positive statements are what we need to combat our negative thinking, but let's avoid becoming Pollyannaish in the process.

Example: "I don't enjoy my job and I'm going to be brave and quit. Then I know I'll be happier." A more rational response to the same situation would be, "I am seriously thinking of leaving the job I don't care for. But before I do, I am going to do my homework and find out what my options are." That's a big difference.

Be sure to educate yourself before you engage in your head talk. You can hardly respect your message if you don't really know what the message is about. The key is making these statements with authority and vigor and repeating them frequently.

Talking to yourself in a healthy, informed, positive manner will motivate you to make intelligent choices, whether eating, exercise, or relationships.

> If you think you can, you can. If you think you can't, you're right.
>
> — Mary Kay Ash

You can pave the way for this new way of thinking by clearing a mental path. Practice in your head. Picture in your head what you will tell yourself under a given set of circumstances. If you are willing to practice without beating on yourself when you fail, you will win this battle and love the results.

As you learn your REBT and listen to people express their feelings, you will be surprised at how people insist on upsetting themselves with their "shoulds" and "musts." While working on this portion of *Living Thin,* I had occasion to spend a few hours with a friend who just returned from a visit with his son and daughter-in-law. The visit turned out to be a miserable one for all concerned. He was critical of the food his daughter-in-law served to his grandchildren and the way she ran her household, and while he truly believes that his feelings are triggered by his love for his son and grandchildren, he fails to realize that his "shoulding" and "musting" serves only to create disharmony.

Some people "get it" in a brief session and others may need intense therapy. Whatever you need, go for it. Moving along in this educational process, which is called "psychotherapy," involves dealing with unhealthy or neurotic thoughts and feelings. However, if you think that once you follow these suggestions you can rid yourself of all emotional disturbances or that you are a neurotic person if you occasionally have a strong emotional reaction, you are so wrong.

Therapists are subject to the same emotions as you and I. The major difference is that they have educated heads. If you do your homework, practice these principles religiously, you, too, can have an educated head.

If you have really worked on these REBT principles and find that they are not working, refuse to give up. Find someone to help you think more clearly, more rationally — someone who will help you to face up to your choices. If you can find someone who practices REBT therapy, that person may also be willing to help you or give you exercises that further your own understanding of these principles.

Whether you find a social worker, peer counselor, or psychiatrist, be sure it is someone you feel comfortable with and who can involve you in the work of becoming a healthier you — an "in charge" you. This is done by making the study and use of the critical thinking skills a part of your life. A good therapist will coach you in the fine art of challenging your irrational beliefs and the thoughts that lead you to feeling upset and powerless, in other words, to make "thinking about thinking" a part of your life.

REBT, Dr. Ellis's approach to therapy, is exciting because it works, and it works within a very short time. Unlike Freudian therapy, which devotes endless hours to discussing and dissecting your past, REBT deals with issues here and now. In a world as fast paced as ours, who has the time, the energy, the dollars to go on and on about a problem that needs repair quickly? REBT is practical and intelligent. It addresses the issue directly, forcing you to address choices almost immediately. Therein lies the magic of REBT.

Buddhism has become popular in America, in part because of its perspective on problem solving. One of the more well-known stories in the Buddhist texts is one that deals with a person shot through the shoulder by an arrow and bleeding profusely. As he is bleeding, people ponder such inane queries as the kind of wood the arrow was made of, where the bow was made, etc. — things that do not help them minister to the injured man at all. The story illustrates nicely how absurd it is to inquire into peripheral and inconsequential facts that do not advance a needed remedy.

Instead, the emphasis in REBT, like Buddhism, is on the present problem, the most suitable and immediate remedy, and ways of preventing it from happening again. Similarly, here are the "rules" for rational living.

SYLVIA'S RATIONAL RULES FOR LIVING THIN

During the many years I have taught Living Thin classes, I kept a record of conversations I had with students who often revealed themselves during the nine-week series. The following rules for rational living evolved from these real-life episodes. Of course, while the stories are true, the names have been changed.

Life Is So Unfair

Marilyn and Madeline were sisters who joined the class, determined to lose weight in time for their younger brother's wedding (a poor reason for making the many changes they needed to make for permanent change). Madeline began losing weight easily, almost effortlessly, while Marilyn struggled and agonized as she discovered that in spite of reducing calories, giving up her favorite desserts, and doubling her exercise, she was losing slowly. Indeed, at times the needle on the scale refused to budge. *"So unfair,"* she lamented. *"My sister cheats, eats sweets, rarely exercises, and yet manages to lose weight easily while I,*

who observe all the rules religiously, am engaged in an extraor-
dinary struggle. Madeline's metabolism is obviously superior to
mine. It's just too unfair."

Life Is Unfair. Good people are often unlucky in love and in life. Mean spirited individuals all too often wind up with "life's goodies." Did anyone ever tell you life is fair? Most people have a pretty fair amount of unfairness during a lifetime. Accepting the fact that Madeline's metabolism allows her to eat more junk foods and lose weight is frustrating, whereas you must exercise caution and need to accept your body's resistance to weight loss. Why not think about the health aspects: her metabolism permits her to eat junk foods that are unhealthy while you are learning healthy eating habits that, in the long run, will pay off in terms of improved health. So life is unfair, and So What! At times that same unfairness can be a plus.

Love Yourself Unconditionally, But Make Yourself Do Hard Things

Mary Jane was forever admiring the achievements of others — rarely giving herself credit for any accomplishment. As she talked her heart out during a few Living Thin classes, we learned that nearly all of her major life choices had been selected for her by others — including a variety of diet programs that left her with more weight and even less self-confidence.

While enrolled in Living Thin, she was encouraged to make her own food and exercise choices. As she began experiencing success in these areas, her self-confidence increased. Very soon she realized she could, indeed, do hard things and didn't need others to make decisions for her. Before the program ended Mary Jane discovered that she was fully capable of making decisions that reflected *her* needs and values — not those of others.

You Can Be the Boss Sometimes, But Not All the Time

Sam worked for a computer company with offices all over the world. Shortly before joining our program he was promoted to marketing director, a position he had dreamed of achieving for many years. Nearly 500 employees assisted him, listened to his ideas, and helped implement his programs. He cherished this power and found himself "living the role" in situations unrelated to his work.

When he joined the Living Thin Program we learned very quickly that he had two major problems:

1. He was a know-it-all. *"I already know all about the importance of nutrition, portion control and exercise, blah, blah, blah."*

   What he needed to learn was that while he may have known a lot, he didn't know it all or he wouldn't have had the problem. He needed to learn how to motivate himself to DO the things he knew needed to be done.

2. His head needed to be educated. He needed to learn how his body responded to various types of food, how much he could eat and how much he would need to exercise in order to lose, maintain, or gain weight.

These principles and guidelines can be found in Chapters 4 and 5, and until and unless you gain this information, you cannot be in charge. Accept this fact: You can be the boss sometime, but until you get the Living Thin education, your body will be the boss.

So You're Not Perfect. So What! Laugh At Your Mistakes

During one class, Christina boasted about her pride in keeping an exquisitely immaculate home at all times. She added that she had trained her family to adhere to her strict standards. She went on to confide that in spite of her passion for perfectionism she could never seem to find a perfect solution for her overweight problem.

I also recall my response: "Well, I'm not surprised to learn about your failure. A major premise of this program is avoiding the need to be perfect — understanding that this quest for perfectionism is a deterrent, a minus, not a plus."

Demanding perfection, especially when you are changing a lifestyle, results in setting unrealistic, unreasonable goals, which often leads to anxiety, which in turn results in your using food to relieve the anxiety. While change is the goal, that change need not be perfect. You can win this battle without being perfect. Give up your demand for achieving a perfect solution. To be perfect means succeeding 100 percent of the time. (I will probably choose to be perfect none of the time.) This perfectionist kind of thinking creates the kind of negative attitude that defeats goals. Pursuing a goal seriously is fine, but taking yourself too seriously is not funny.

How Much You Weigh Doesn't Define Who You Are

Terry had a difficult time accepting the unalterable fact that she would never, ever, regardless of the year or occasion, wear a Size 6 garment. Her bones, her genetics, her nature made it obvious that her goal was unrealistic and completely irrational.

However, she doesn't have to wear a size 20. With effort and practice she can wear 12s and look as fashionable as anyone wearing a size 6. Because she was most willing, even eager, to pay her dues and do what she needed to do to lose and maintain her weight, we encouraged Terry to respect and accept this attitude, which is intelligent and reasonable.

Being overweight means nothing more or less than being overweight. It doesn't say anything about your values, the quality of your work, your sense of humor, your personality, or the way you make love. Refuse to feel uncomfortable about your weight. As long as you're in the game, you'll feel good about yourself. Avoid insisting on 100 percent success.

Living Involves Some Form of Hassle Every Single Day

Rachel loved the real estate business. She started her own business as a young person and became one of the most important and successful people in her field. From the beginning of her career she trained herself to accept the inevitable frustrations and disappointments connected with sales.

During the nine weeks of the Living Thin Program she described a variety of situations that produced extreme stress, always resulting in binges. The major issue became why she was unable to apply her attitude skills to frustrating issues unrelated to her business.

Rachel finally realized the problem stemmed from an unwillingness to apply herself seriously to any task not connected with her business. We finally persuaded her to examine the consequences of her indifference to health issues. When she began applying the same common sense thinking to health matters that had become second nature to her in her real estate business, the program worked and she lost weight.

A day without hassles is a rare day.

Happiness Involves Effort and Action

Happiness and self-sufficiency are compatible companions. They go hand in hand. They belong together. Children characteristically look to others to take care of their needs, but adults find that being happy is difficult when we insist on depending on others for our happiness.

Finally, the essence of *Living* Thin — not *Getting* Thin: Growing up and accepting responsibility for making your own choices — including controlling your weight and your response to life's hassles. BEING IN CHARGE TASTES BETTER THAN A HOT FUDGE SUNDAE!

WHAT TO DO WHEN

Here are several typical scenarios we commonly face and how to use rational thinking to stay on track and reach your goals.

You Are Doing Everything Right
and It Still Isn't Working

A. SITUATION

I am using the Living Thin blueprint and it still isn't working to take off any pounds. I use the chart, count my calories as suggested, but I am not losing weight.

B. IN YOUR HEAD

1. "This is terrible. I cannot and will not eat less than I am now consuming."
2. "I've given up ice cream and sweets."
3. "I can't stand being this fat. I hate it. I hate it."

C. FEELINGS

Depressed, very upset.

D. QUESTION YOUR HEAD TALK

Remember what Chapter 2 says: "It is not the situation that causes your upsettedness but rather what you are telling yourself in your head about the situation.

Challenge your head talk:

1. *"Not losing weight is hardly terrible as long as it is not causing any acute health problems."*
2. *"Yes, it is disappointing and discouraging. But before I decide that I will never wear a size 12, why not examine my eating chart and try to discover why the needle on the scale is not moving."*
3. *"It is important to understand and accept the fact that weight loss is scientific for everyone; my friends, my enemies, and me. When I consume 3500 calories less than my body requires to maintain its present weight, I will lose about one pound of fat."*
4. *"Am I sure I am counting correctly, not fibbing on my chart?"*

I have found that people often kid themselves about what and how much they are eating and then feel depressed about it when it isn't working.

E. CHOICES

1. Examine your chart carefully. Avoid fibbing and use this as an opportunity to learn about calories and yourself.

2. Look for sodium content in foods that may be causing you to retain water.
3. Find a "diet" that will give you what you want without any responsibility on your part.
4. Give up.
5. Accept the information you are learning and work around it.

It is important, however, to understand and accept the scientific data about weight loss. By following your Living Thin guidelines outlined in Chapters 4 and 5 you will understand these principles. If you are doing what you need to do but are failing to lose weight, then you clearly are not ready to accept the message. And that's OK. Refuse to upset yourself. Wait until you are ready to work harder at doing the things you need to do.

Life Rains on Your Parade In a Big Way

A. SITUATION

Other issues have arisen in my life and I no longer care to make the effort to Live Thin. My husband has just left me for a young, attractive, intelligent, and wealthy woman. I cannot possibly compete with her, and my only solace is EATING.

B. IN YOUR HEAD

1. *"I will be alone the rest of my life. I will never find another partner."*
2. *"How dare he leave me when I was such a devoted and loving wife!"*

3. *"What a fool I am. I gave up so many things to please him."*

4. *"Giving up my favorite food at this point in my life is horrible — much too difficult."*

C. FEELINGS

Angry, depressed, upset.

D. QUESTION YOUR HEAD TALK

It is not the situation that causes your upsettedness but rather what you are telling yourself in your head about the situation.

Challenge your head talk:

1. *"There is no guarantee I will be alone. However, if I insist on gaining more weight and walk around depressed, I have a pretty good chance of living alone."*

2. *"He dares because he dares. Of course I am upset. It is natural; who wouldn't be in my position? But he doesn't need my permission to behave this way. In fact, he has the right to choose to do these things regardless of how cruel it seems to me and our children. Why should he live with me if what he wants is to live with another person?"*

3. *"What I did may or may not have influenced his actions."*

4. *"While I may never like it, accepting it will make it easier to live with."*

5. *"It may be difficult but think of the consequences. Will eating recklessly improve my situation or will it add to my despondency and worries?"*

E. CHOICES

1. Accept what happened and make plans to get on with your life.

2. Begin thinking in terms of your health and appearance and become a role model for your children.

3. Wail and whine and eat yourself into oblivion.

4. Give up.

You Are Losing
Motivation and Commitment

A. SITUATION

I am tired, bored, weary of thinking and planning to reverse a lifetime of habits. In spite of my respect for this approach, I am feeling deprived.

B. IN YOUR HEAD

1. *"I can't stand the idea of thinking and planning. Neither can I stand the idea of regaining my weight."*

2. *"This is terrible. I have devoted so much time to making it work and losing some weight. There must be something wrong with me."*

C. FEELINGS

Frustrated, depressed, very upset.

D. QUESTION YOUR HEAD TALK

It is not the situation that causes your upsettedness but rather what you are telling yourself in your head about the situation.

Challenge your head talk:

1. *"I can stand the thinking and planning. I am simply bored."*
2. *"It's not terrible, it's just disappointing."*
3. *"How silly to say there is something wrong with me. Reversing a lifetime of eating habits is tough and I am not alone."*

E. CHOICES

1. Think about how willing you are to revamp your eating choices. You can have whatever you choose as long as you are willing to pay the price, perhaps to allow yourself a weekly indulgence. You then have something to look forward to.
2. Choose to reach your goal more slowly. Losing slowly is better than giving up. (There is a huge difference between telling yourself you can "never" eat such and such as opposed to giving yourself the freedom to indulge on occasion.)
3. Give up.

The choices are yours!

TIPS FOR NOT BECOMING A DIET PROGRAM CASUALTY

You have seen them all and tried too many. Don't become a diet program casualty. Here is my short list of warning signs about "popular" diet programs.

1. If it sounds like magic — forget it!

2. If it promises quick weight loss — forget it!

Crash diets promote water and lean tissue loss, which slows down your metabolism. The sad part is that when you regain the weight — and you will — you do not regain muscle; you gain fat. As a result, when you decide to diet again, you will have to eat even less to lose weight because the fat you've added by dieting causes your body to metabolize more slowly.

I would ask new students approximately how many calories they could eat and not gain weight. There was quite a range. For women, between 900 and 1800. I finally learned that those who could consume about 1600–1800 calories had perhaps cut back on what they ate but never dieted. Those who had low caloric intakes (approximately 900–1100) were having difficulty not gaining. They were telling me, without realizing it, that they had been on numerous crash diets and had slowed down their metabolism by their dieting. Their crash dieting had "trained" their bodies to make do with less, and they were still having trouble maintaining a suitable weight! The message comes through loud and clear: The intelligent solution is: LONG-TERM WEIGHT LOSS CAN'T BE ACCOMPLISHED BY CRASH DIETS. Accept this or accept the consequences.

3. While you are learning to make healthy lifestyle choices, be sure these choices are compatible with your tastes, habits, and preferences.

TACTICS FOR SUCCESS

1. No food is forbidden.

Does that shock you? Let me explain. If I say you cannot have cookies, cake, and ice cream, all you will think about is cookies, cake, and ice cream.

Let's say you've given up heavy duty sweets like pie à la mode for six months and think that indulging on occasion won't matter. It won't matter, provided you've really overcome your addiction to sweets. If, however, you are still in love with, and addicted to sweets, you may tell yourself that you can handle it.

Then, before too long you enter the sweet zone again and when you do, your chances for keeping it off are kaput — GONE. I am not suggesting that you cannot enjoy a milk shake (about 650 calories) once in a while. Even a very rich snack will never cause you to gain more than a pound or so.

What I am saying is be sure you are over your addiction. It's the same with old flames — be sure you have gotten over them before you see them again. And remember, be willing to compromise, if you can't have Tom, take Harry. If you can't have chocolate cheesecake, have chocolate nonfat yogurt.

Knowing how to get back on track instead of giving up is more important than having a "must" or a "never" in your head. And refuse to wail and whine when you find yourself having a difficult time getting back on track. It *is* difficult. So What? Not getting back on track is more difficult.

All I am saying is that you should not become rigid and restrained about your food choices.

Do your best to include foods you enjoy even if they cost you a little more and even if they slow down the weight loss process. Developing an eating plan you find enjoyable as well as healthy is the basis for your Living Thin lifestyle.

2. The day you start your eating chart is the day you begin changing your eating habits.

Keep it on your fridge and keep it filled in. You will have to jot down eating notes during the day. I don't believe in complicated eating journals. Chapters 4 and 5 tell you all you need to know about keeping track.

3. Choose no more than one or two changes a week.

For example: In one week you can commit to walking three times and being more assertive with your mother-in-law. Trying to do everything at once will cause you to feel frustrated and overwhelmed. Avoid moving on to new areas until you feel the habit you are working on has taken hold.

4. Identify times and situations when you are vulnerable to overeating.

For instance, you may be more apt to overeat when you are angry, bored, or stressed. Review Chapter 3.

5. Think calories.

The case for and against calories has been raging for more than 100 years. And here is the answer:

Many influential people in health professions have decided to capitalize on the weight issue and the public's refusal to use calorie counting by telling you that "fat and protein are in" and that "carbohydrates are out." When we fail as a society to deal effectively and healthily with reversing overweight, the professionals blame the public rather than finding fault with their theory. The same thing happens when calorie counting is "in" and fails to do the job due to a failure to correctly understand and use the principles involved. It goes back and forth with one constant: many people are making tons of money and the rest are failing to lose tons of unhealthy pounds.

The same rules apply to calories as to money. By that I mean you cannot spend money you don't have without going into debt, and you cannot consume more calories than you can afford without gaining weight. This is what is meant by saying "weight loss is scientific."

However, there are important differences in the way your body metabolizes carbohydrates (pasta, grain, fruit, bread) and the way your body processes proteins (fish, chicken, beef) and fats/oils. You need to educate yourself about the differences and base your food choices on your knowledge of the subject *as it applies to your situation.*

Carbohydrates do cost more because they metabolize more slowly. So while you are trying to lose weight, remember these facts about carbohydrates. But don't give them up, otherwise you are back to "dieting." Simply reduce your intake.

The overriding issue is about making your own choices. Otherwise it won't work. At times you will be eating more carbohydrates and at others more protein. What determines your long-term success is that your decisions are YOURS — that is Living Thin.

6. Parties — Giving Them — Going to Them

a. See yourself declining food offers. The clearer the picture in your head, the easier it will be to do it.

b. Eat a small snack before going to a party (or out to dinner). This will subdue your appetite.

c. When you arrive at a party or restaurant, do a little window shopping to get an idea of how you can eat to match how you want to feel when you leave.

d. Include or exclude alcohol, but plan it in advance. Adding a no-calorie mixer like mineral water or diet tonic water will make your drink go much further.

e. During the cocktail hour, train yourself to limit yourself to one, two (or none) hors d'oeuvres. Concentrate instead on conversation. A major achievement!

f. Practice being assertive when you accept or reject food or drink.

7. Daily Reminders

a. When you shop, purchase only what is on your list.

b. If you cannot avoid nibbling while preparing food, make sure you have a "nibble bowl" of vegetables to get you to mealtime.

c. Think about and plan to enjoy a variety of foods every day. Try new foods.

d. Get on the scale every day. If your weight goes up, think about your eating from the previous day that may have caused water retention (cola drinks or salty foods are culprits here).

e. Refuse to get upset.

f. Plan to eat at least five times a day.

g. Get some exercise every day. It can be as little as 3–5 minutes. Doing it every day, forming the habit is the goal.

h. Have a food plan every day.

Doing it this way is really the easy way. The hard way is to fight it and look to others to do it for you.

FREQUENTLY ASKED QUESTIONS

1. *I'm doing all the right things: exercising, cutting my calories, giving up desserts, giving up cocktails (this person really believes what he or she is saying) and I'm not losing weight. What should I do?*

The first thing to do is stop lying! Review the information about weight loss being scientific. When you consume 3500 calories less than the body needs to maintain its present weight, your body will shed one pound — unless you are having a water retention problem, which could result from a menstrual period or consuming ingredients such as sodium or MSG. Some medications, such as Prednisone also cause water retention.

2. *How do I get back on track after I spent the weekend overeating?*

Getting back on track is like dancing — the best way to learn how to dance is to dance. Recognize that you have an attitude problem. Refuse to give up on yourself. Refuse to feel guilty. Whip out that eating chart and respect it. Honor it. And start again. If in the past you messed up frequently and you are now messing up infrequently, that is considered progress.

I'd like to hear from you. Your feedback will help me determine what you liked best and what you liked least and where your interests lie. Write me at the following address: 2450 Harbourside Drive, #252, Longboat Key, Florida 34228.

CONCLUSION

This book is an affirmation.

It is about attitudes, health, change, being overweight, and youthful aging. Being overweight in America often means being confused, powerless, frustrated, self-conscious and anxious about the most important part of your life — Your Health.

It is also a primer on taking control of the misguided ship many overweight Americans are aboard. Overweight Americans are not only unhealthy, they are deceived and exploited by the weight loss industry, which succeeds when you fail to be in control of your own eating and exercise programs, your own education, and your own emotions. In other words — your life.

Living Thin, Living Young began as a protest against dieting and ended up as a preventive health program that will result in healthy aging. Living Thin (not Getting Thin) involves nutrition, exercise, and stress control — a trio that becomes the core of preventive medicine. And preventive medicine will slow down the aging process. Using the principles in this book will help you set goals to assume responsibility for your own health — so you, too, can enjoy "Living Thin, Living Young." Enjoy the journey!

NOTES

Chapter 2

1. Paul Hauck, *How To Do What You Want To Do: The Art of Self-Discipline,* Philadelphia: The Westminster Press, 1976, p. 12.

Chapter 3

1. David Hungerford, M.D., from a video made in the home of author, 1991.
2. David Reuben, M.D., *Everything You Always Wanted To Know About Nutrition,* New York: Simon & Schuster, 1978, pp. 17–18.

Chapter 4

1. Jack Osman, Ph.D., *Fat . . . Fat . . . Fat,* Towson, Maryland: Fat Control, Inc., 1984, p. 91.

Chapter 5

1. Gaylord Hauser, *Mirror, Mirror on the Wall, Invitation to Beauty,* New York: Farrar, Straus and Cudahy, 1960, pp. 151–154.
2. Ibid.
3. Gaylord Hauser, *Gaylord Hauser's Treasury of Secrets,* New York: Farrar, Straus and Company, 1951, pp. 381–382.
4. Harvey and Marilyn Diamond, *Fit for Life II,* New York: Warner Books, 1987, p. 29.
5. John Yudkin, M.D., *Sweet and Dangerous,* New York: Peter H. Wyden, Inc., 1972, p. 3.
6. Robert C. Atkins, M.D., *Dr. Atkins' Health Revolution,* New York: Bantam, 1990, p. 87.
7. Nancy Appleton, Ph.D., *Lick the Sugar Habit,* New York: Avery Publishing Group, 1996, p. 1.
8. William Dufty, *Sugar Blues,* Radmor, Pennsylvania: Chilton Book Co., 1975, p. 69.

Bibliography

Barnard, Neal, M.D. *Food for Life, How the New Four Food Groups Can Save Your Life.* New York: Crown. 1993.

Brody, Jane. *Jane Brody's Nutrition Book.* New York: W. W. Norton & Co., 1981.

Diamond, Harvey and Marilyn. *Fit for Life.* New York: Warner Books. 1985.

Diamond, Harvey and Marilyn. *Fit for Life II.* New York: Warner Books. 1987.

Ellis, Albert, Ph.D., *How to Stubbornly Refuse to Make Yourself Miserable About Anything, Yes Anything.* New York: Carol Communications. 1988.

Ellis, Albert, Ph.D., and Emmett Velten, Ph.D., *Optimal Aging, Get Over Getting Older.* Chicago: Open Court. 1998.

Irons, Diane. *The World's Best-Kept Diet Secrets.* Naperville, IL: Sourcebooks, Inc. 1998.

Jakubowski, Patricia, and Arthur J. Lange. *The Assertive Option, Your Rights & Responsibilities.* Champaign, IL: Lange Research Press Company. 1978.

Null, Gary, Ph.D., *Gary Null's Ultimate Anti-Aging Program.* New York: Kensington Books. 1999.

Roizen, Michael F., M.D., *Real Age, Are You As Young As You Can Be?* New York: Cliff Street Books. 1999.

The following books are recommended for other recipes:

Brody, Jane. *Jane Brody's Good Food Book*. New York: W. W. Norton & Co., 1985.

Snyder, Hinman. *Lean and Luscious*, Vol. I and II. Rocklin, CA: Prima Publishing & Communications. 1987, 1988.

Newsletters

Nutrition Action Health Letter
Center for Science in the Public Interest
1875 Connecticut Ave., N.W. Suite 300, Washington, DC 20009

Prescriptions for Healthy Living
Weiss Research
4176 Burns Rd.
Palm Beach Gardens, Florida 33410

Women's Health Advisor
Torstar Publications, Inc.
99 Hawley Lane
Stratford, CT 06614

Catalog of Books, Study Aids

Institute for Rational-Emotive Therapy
45 East 65th Street
New York, NY 10021-6593

Index

Aggression, 11, 201, 205, 206, 218, 228, 237
Aging, 107, 119, 135, 138, 165, 176, 250, 288
Alcoholic, 24, 27, 106, 126, 133
Anger, 43
Antiobesity pills, 62
Anxiety, 43
Appleton, Nancy, Ph.D.
 Lick the Sugar Habit, 154
Arthritis, 163, 168, 169, 170, 171, 251
Assert, 201, 203, 204, 205, 207, 226, 228, 240, 241, 245
Assertiveness, 201, 218, 219, 220, 229, 230, 231, 237, 240, 241
Attitude, 27, 33, 40, 67, 68, 70, 71, 72, 88, 132, 159, 172, 174, 189, 192, 221, 225, 243, 250, 253, 259, 274, 275, 287
Autotoxicity, 148
Awfulizing, 42, 48

Behaviorists, 223
Bingeing, 126, 128, 130, 131
Body language, 220

Boredom, 19, 34, 77, 86, 96
Breakfast, necessity of eating, 84
Breakfasts, 142
Brody, Jane, 165

Calories, 3, 4, 23, 33, 35, 57, 63, 67, 75, 86, 87, 89, 98ff, 108ff, 116ff, 140, 142, 143, 144, 146, 156, 158, 159, 164, 165, 167, 175, 177 - 187, 192, 196, 210, 243 - 245, 263, 268, 271, 276, 277, 282 - 285, 287
 by food classification, 105
 getting more pleasure, 118
Carbohydrates, 120, 121, 140, 142, 143, 285
Change, difficulties of, 83
Chocolate, 125
Cleave, T. L.,
 The SaccharineDisease, 153
Cocktails, 32, 117, 151, 257, 287
Commitment, 7, 14, 15, 18, 39, 94, 157, 200, 207, 246
Compulsive eating, 132
Compulsive nature, author's, 256

Dairy products, 120, 145
Depression, 24, 41, 44, 45, 55, 63, 81,
    87, 115, 166, 167, 170, 172, 189,
    200, 203, 214, 251, 254, 267
Desserts, 74, 126, 211, 271, 287
Dewey, John, 13
Diet groups, 3
Diet mentality
    freeing you from, 118
Diet, Banana and Skim Milk, 3
Dietitian, 1, 4
Diets are for Dummies, 69
Diets don't work, 2, 12
Diets, why they fail, 249
Dufty, William, 155
    The Sugar Blues, 155

Eating chart, 65, 66, 67, 76, 85, 101,
    115, 131, 132, 189, 233, 238, 246,
    256, 258, 259, 260, 277, 284, 287
Eating more and weighing less, 114
Eating on the run, 89, 95
Edison, Thomas, 33
Elimination, 22, 144, 145, 147, 150
Elizabeth Taylor, 33, 77
Ellis, Dr. Albert Ellis, 8, 28, 211
Emotional eating, 24
Emotional health, 258
Excuses, 7, 11, 37, 85, 90, 93, 94, 95,
    96, 107, 146, 160, 163, 170, 223,
    251, 263
Exercise, 1, 22, 23, 37, 38, 49, 63, 76,
    86, 87, 95, 96, 98, 108, 114, 115,
    128, 130, 133, 139, 160, 162, 163,
    164, 165, 166, 167, 168, 169, 170,
    171, 172, 173, 174, 189, 191, 211,
    221, 225, 233, 242, 250, 251, 252,
    253, 255, 256, 261, 263, 266, 269,
    271, 272, 273, 286, 288

Fat, 11, 12, 15, 33, 39, 69, 71, 84, 89,
    99, 101, 105, 106, 118, 119, 121,
    122, 123, 124, 127, 137, 139, 140,

    141, 144, 147, 148, 150, 152, 155,
    159, 162, 165, 166, 178, 179, 187,
    210, 252, 276, 277, 282, 284
Fat Foods, 121
Fatigue, 19, 86, 96, 198
Fats, 21, 96, 124, 142, 285
Fear of displeasing others, 207
Fear of hurting others' feelings, 217
Fear of rejection in social situations,
    216
Flies, 159
Frequently asked questions, 287
Fruits, 145, 155
Frustration, 44

Gaby, Dr. Alan, 151
Garbage in your head, 19, 59, 61, 67,
    174
Genetic predisposition, 38
Genetics, 107
Getting started. *See* Exercise
Goals, limit, 39
Goals, realistic, 85, 190
Grains, 120, 142, 145
Grandiosity, 77. *See* Little-King
    Syndrome
Guide to Rational Living, A. See Ellis,
    Dr. Albert
Guilt, 35, 39, 44, 104, 127, 164, 172,
    190, 200, 214, 266, 267, 268
Guilt, refuse to feel guilty, 94

Habit, 40, 154, 189
Hauck, Dr. Paul, 36, 226
Hauser, 135, 137, 138, 141, 142
Hauser, Gaylord
    Mirror, Mirror, On The Wall, 135
Hauser, Gaylord, 135, 138, 140, 141
Hauserman-Campbell, Dr. Norma, 7, 8,
    229
Head talk, 51, 53, 73, 76, 87, 88, 89,
    91, 93, 96, 189, 213, 214, 215, 223,
    236, 238, 254, 268, 277, 279, 281

Health
  becoming an absolute snob about,
    144
Health and nutrition, attitudes, 70
Healthy Weight Journal. See Levitsky,
  David
Hillel, Rabbi, 221
*How to Do What You Want To Do: The
  Art of Self-Discipline. See* Hauck,
  Dr. Paul
Humiliation, 44

Junk foods, 73, 221, 272

Klinefelter, Dr. Harry, 8

Legumes, 120, 145
Levitsky, David, 62
LFT — Low Frustration Tolerance, 12,
  13, 18, 19, 34, 72, 74, 75, 76, 77,
  133,134, 254
Little-King Syndrome, 77
Living Assertively, 200
Living Thin Program, 1, 2, 8, 13, 23,
  59, 60, 142, 193, 213, 256, 273, 275
Loneliness, 77
Low-calorie, 57, 65, 99, 141

Meal Plans, 177
Mental Jogging. *See* Self-talk
Metabolism, 12, 38, 63, 107, 108, 140,
  142, 143, 164, 243, 272, 282
Mind-body reactions to negative self-
  talk, 267
Mood swings, 172
Motivation, 11, 15, 19, 31, 40, 59, 60,
  62, 76, 78, 79, 80, 81, 82, 83, 84,
  85, 86, 96, 168, 193, 198, 203, 204,
  207, 236, 246, 254, 280
Motivation, wrong kind, 82

Nibbling, 124, 125, 126
Niebuhr, Reinhold, 259

Nutritionist, become your own, 250

Oetinger, Friedrich, 259
Orwell, George
  Animal Farm, 119
Osman, Dr. Jack, 7, 99,140, 156
Overweights, 26, 84, 95, 98, 152, 164,
  250, 263

Parties, giving them, going to them,
  285
Penalty and reward system, 86
Permanent connection groups, 247
Planning, 23, 24, 188, 189, 190, 191,
  192, 196
Planning, fear of, 23
Polaner's jelly, 144, 158
Portion control, 21
Positive statements, 268
Power struggles, 36
Priorities, 86, 191, 229, 258
Procrastination, 86
Protein foods, 119

Rational rules for living thin, 271
Rational thinking, 11, 27, 28, 41, 42,
  47, 50, 55, 59, 84, 89, 133, 193,
  200, 213, 238, 242, 253, 258, 259,
  267, 276
Rationality in an irrational world, 26
Real foods, 39
REBT, 7, 8, 28, 31, 41, 45, 47, 48, 51,
  55, 58, 59, 91, 93, 193, 211, 226,
  238, 253, 260, 269, 270, 271
Relationships, 82, 228
Restaurants, 243
Reuben, David, M.D., 70
Ridgidity
  avoiding it, 115
Risk taking, 237
Rowe, John, M.D., and Robert Kahn,
  Ph.D. *Successful Aging*, 138

Salad, 110, 111, 112, 114, 116, 122, 123, 126, 142, 143, 146, 183, 184, 185, 186, 245
Salt, 21, 22, 96, 121, 143, 144, 148, 197
Sedentary living, 164
Self-Acceptance, 14, 93, 232, 255
Self-Confidence, 57, 233
Self-discipline, 8, 31, 32, 33, 34, 36, 37, 38, 79, 192, 262
Self-downing, 255
Self-esteem, 58, 62, 75, 84, 192, 202, 232, 246, 254, 267
Self-talk, 74, 85, 87, 91, 92, 93, 94, 95, 168, 198, 213, 266, 267
Shaw, Dr. Buzz, 232
Shaw, Dr. Kenneth, 7
Skinner, B. F., 28
Slender people, 39, 92, 99, 118, 119, 127, 210
Smith, Dr. Lendon, 154
Smoking, 3
Snack and Dessert Choices, 144
Snickers bar, 123
Soup, 39, 103, 112, 117, 143, 180, 182, 185, 245
Soup, noncream-based, 143
Stevia, 158
Stinking thinking, 8, 19, 36, 46, 50, 68, 84, 87, 89, 96, 236, 266
Stoic, become a, 40
Stress, 9, 29, 58, 59, 60, 63, 96, 134, 140, 175, 176, 188, 191, 242, 246, 249, 255, 267, 275, 288
Sugar, 45, 70, 89, 92, 96, 109, 110, 112, 120, 133, 141, 142, 150, 151, 152, 153, 154, 155, 156, 157, 158, 159, 160, 198
Sugarholic, 150

Tactics for success, 283
Thin From Within. See Osman, Dr. Jack
Time, not enough of it, 242
Toxins, 145, 149
Two-year-old-ism, 76

Upsettedness, 41, 89, 189, 200, 239, 258, 260, 265, 277, 279, 281

Vegetables, 107

Water, 15, 38, 106, 117, 123, 125, 142, 143, 146, 147, 148, 149, 150, 166, 167, 177, 178, 179, 180, 181, 182, 183, 184, 185, 186, 187, 197, 244, 278, 282, 286, 287
 connection to weight loss, health, and aging, 146
Weight control, 1, 41, 59, 151
Weight loss, 4, 5, 7, 8, 9, 11, 12, 13, 24, 27, 32, 33, 35, 39, 62, 63, 65, 67, 68, 71, 72, 77, 80, 85, 92, 98, 99, 100, 102, 103, 108, 115, 119, 120, 138, 139, 141, 143, 144, 146, 147, 150, 156, 164, 167, 172, 174, 175, 188, 204, 210, 211, 246, 249, 250, 255, 256, 261, 263, 264, 272, 277, 278, 282, 283, 285, 287, 288
 personal prescription, 108
Weight loss industry, 5, 72, 288
Weight loss is scientific, 4
Weight loss or maintanence, Sylvia's prescription, 116
Weight loss, easy answers, 9
Wine. *See* calories
Wooley, Monte, 70

Yogurt, 106, 142, 144, 158, 182, 187, 283
Yudkin, Dr. John, 152 - 154